A Dialogue

on Love

Also by Eve Kosofsky Sedgwick

The Coherence of Gothic Conventions
Between Men: English Literature and Male Homosocial Desire
Epistemology of the Closet
Tendencies
Fat Art, Thin Art

Edited by Eve Kosofsky Sedgwick

Shame and Its Sisters: A Silvan Tomkins Reader (*coeditor*)
Gary in Your Pocket: Stories and Notebooks of Gary Fisher
Performativity and Performance (*coeditor*)
Novel Gazing: Queer Readings in Fiction

Eve Kosofsky

Sedgwick

A Dialogue
on Love

Beacon Press

Boston

Beacon Press

25 Beacon Street

Boston, Massachusetts 02108-2892

www.beacon.org

Beacon Press books

are published under the auspices of

the Unitarian Universalist Association

of Congregations.

© 1999 by Eve Kosofsky Sedgwick

Printed in the United States of America

06 05 04 03 02 01 00   9 8 7 6 5 4 3 2

Excerpt of "The Kimono" from *Selected Poems 1946–1985* by James Merrill. Copyright ©1992 by James Merrill. Reprinted by permission of Alfred A. Knopf, Inc.

Excerpt of "The Book of Ephraim" from *The Changing Light at Sandover* by James Merrill. Copyright ©1980, 1982 by James Merrill. Reprinted by permission of Alfred A. Knopf, Inc.

This book is printed on acid-free
paper that meets the uncoated
paper ANSI/NISO specifications
for permanence as revised in 1992.

Library of Congress Cataloging-in-Publication Data can be found on page 222.

Thank you, Shannon. Tim, thanks! And I thank my precious family, my friends.

A Dialogue

on Love

1992

Apparently it's as a patient that I want to emerge. "Oh, I guess I'm supposed to call you my client, not my patient," Shannon said once, "but that's the way they taught us, back in graduate school—seems like too much trouble to change."

Besides, I like "patient." It is true I can be very patient. And Shannon is like this too, so the word doesn't feel like placing me at a distance. Then, it seems a modest

> word that makes no claim
> to anything but—wanting
> to be happier

and wanting, it's true, someone else to shoulder a lot of agency in the matter of my happiness.

———————

The day after I left my message, the phone offered a friendly, masculine voice with some

> hard midwestern sounds.
> Eve Sedgwick? Shannon Van Wey.
> *Oh!* Maybe I'm found?

And then in the waiting room, do I have a mental image of him at all? The handsome, lean, well-dressed therapists female and male in this large practice filter through the sunny room, greeting their patients, ushering them up or across . . .

I look expectantly at each of the men.

And I'm trying now to remember it, the grotesque, reassuring shock of Shannon hovering down a few stairs into this view, mild and bristling with his soft gray nap,

> big-faced, cherubic—
> barrel chest, long arms, short legs,
> Rumpelstiltskin-like

and wearing, I've no doubt, a beautifully ironed

> short-sleeved cotton shirt
> the color of an after-
> dinner mint, tucked in

at his rotund waist. If it was as hot as Durham usually is in early September, he had a handkerchief too for mopping his forehead.

There would have been a substantial rumble of genial introduction. My tentative greeting maybe not quite audible in the middle of it. Was this ordinary for him—the first encounter in this familiar room with big, female, middle-aged bodies deprecated by the softness of our voices? Maybe in some manual it's the secret definition of "depression."

And yet (I told him, settled in his office upstairs), it's not so clear to me that "depressed" is the right word for what I am. Depressed is

> what everyone says—
> I'm weeping in a lot of
> offices these days

(and I'm sure the tears slipped over my lids as I said it). But I think I *know* depression, I have my own history of it; and it felt, twenty years ago when I really was subject to it, so much less bearable than this does. So much.

"And yet, you're crying now."

———

In an expensively renovated old building, a space. A large, rugless square made almost cubic by its lofty ceiling. The low bookcases hold not overly many books; the low desk shows a modest, tractable paper mess; framed prints, in a few neat sheaves on the floor, look as if they could wait years more for hanging.

Under the tall windows there's a scattering of the meaningful chotchkas that I suppose people give their shrinks—many are made of glass. Big chairs flank a sofa bland with patches of pastel.

Space not only light with sun and canister lighting but, if there's an appreciative way to use the word, "lite," metaphysically lite. I'm wondering

whether it reflects
no personality, or
already is one.

———

On record, the triggering event was a breast cancer diagnosis eighteen months ago.

Shannon doesn't produce an empathetic face at this, or say "That must have been hard for you." He makes an economical nod.

"I kind of did beautifully with it. I bounced back from the mastectomy, and when it turned out that there was some lymph node involvement too, I tolerated six months of chemotherapy without too many side effects. You know, I *hated* it, and it completely wore me down, but . . .

"The saving thing was that for me it wasn't all about dread. I know there are people whose deepest dread is to have cancer, to undergo surgery, to deal with the likelihood of dying." I shake my head many times.

Those are not my deepest dread. I dread

every bad thing
that threatens people I love;
for me, dread only

I may stop knowing
how to like and desire
the world around me.

"That's it, what you mean by real depression?"

"Oh, yeah."

In some ways the cancer diagnosis came at the best possible time. —The best time if feeling ready to die is a criterion. It was about two months after a book of mine had come out.

"What kind of books do you write?"

I tell Shannon I'm a literary critic; I work in gay and lesbian studies.

The book was *Epistemology of the Closet*, and the writing, the organization of it had came very hard to me for some reason. "So I was amazed at how satisfying its publication was. As an object, the book itself looked lovely—everyone said so. And for an academic book it got a lot of attention, a lot of praise.

"It was one of those happy times when you say to yourself, Okay, this is good, this is enough; I'm ready to go now. When the diagnosis came I was feeling—as an intellectual—loved, used, appreciated. I would have been very, very content to quit while I was ahead."

"Did it surprise you to be feeling that?"

"No. No."

No.

To feel loved and appreciated—I've slowly grown used to that. And to feel the wish of not living! It's one of the oldest sensations I can remember.

————————

"But you didn't get your wish."

"Oh, no, breast cancer doesn't usually work like that. I *felt* sick, but that was from the treatment, not the illness—if the cancer ever does get me, it probably won't be for years. And the chances of that are something like fifty-fifty."

Probably there's a smile on Shannon's face after I produce this. Certainly not because he wants me sick, and not either because he's glad I could be well. It's because, momentarily, he identifies with the mechanical elegance of the trap this disease has constructed for an anxious and ambivalent psyche. Fifty-fifty, I think he's thinking: perfect for turning this particular person inside out.

Sometime in these early sessions, Shannon says about why he became a therapist: "I've always been fascinated by machines. When I was a kid, I'd take them apart and put them back together just to make sure I knew how they worked. It's still a lot of the reason I like my job."

First encounter: my
therapist's gift for guyish
banalization.

————————

I'm forty-two, and what is it I bring to this meeting in the way of expectations? My history as a patient is like my history as a smoker: I tried it a lot of times years ago, but never learned to inhale. All that depression in my teens and twenties means that over the years I've started a lot of therapy. Especially in the hardest years, in graduate school, there were several attempts to get shrunk, one lasting an entire six months. They all ran aground in the same way. I'd go to these women (women, of course: I was a woman, and who else could understand

> if not another
> woman?) bursting out of my
> eyesockets with pain

and within three or four sessions at most, a particular impasse would have gotten wedged so firmly between us we could neither of us move.

Shannon is interrogative.

"I can't remember well," I say, "and in fact I don't want to, but it always involved the charge of 'intellectualizing.' A typical thing would be for me to say something like, 'I'm not angry, I'm just confused about this-or-that theoretical aspect of the situation,' and for her to respond, 'Then why are both of your hands balled up in fists?' And of course they would be. Can I remember how that makes an impasse? . . ."

. . . Well, I'm sure it's true that I'm not what anyone would call in touch with my feelings. "And in these hideously stylized scenes the woman would demand that I *stop thinking* and start *telling her my feelings* instead. Now as far as I can tell, I don't even have what are normally called feelings! I was being as honest as I could. There was no way to respond to the demand—I hated it—I just felt battered. After a lot of that, it would be only a matter of time till the depression let up ever so little, and I'd realize the therapy hour felt even more punishing than the rest of the week.

"So I'd finally get decisive and quit therapy. And it would always end with the same scene: a woman, suddenly riveted by my severity, wondering to me, 'Why couldn't you have been this way all along?'"

"And do you think you *were* intellectualizing?"

"Oh, I don't know! It was a long time ago, I was in very brittle shape, and I really might have been. But will you think I'm crazy if I say, I don't think I do it very much now?"

"No. It's funny, I don't think so either. I've been listening for it too, and—well, intellectualizing is a real specific kind of defense, it has its own sound to it. Not this sound, so far."

I may even know a little about where it's gone.

I'm thinking, there were some things that happened in the past few years that I had no defenses at all to deal with. It was like the Maginot Line: I marshaled the formidable, practiced resources of the decades-long war of attrition I'd fought with my depressiveness—and they were completely irrelevant. Instantly shattered to bits.

So I think I may have made a near-conscious decision a year ago, after the chemo was over, when my hair was growing back. If I can fit the pieces of this self back together at all, I don't want them to be the way they were. Not because I thought I could be better defended, either: what I wanted was to be realer. What I fear now is

> to have long to thirst
> anymore in the stony
> desert of that self

threatening to recompose itself in the same way in the same dazed and laborious place.

Shannon's interested in this. "You're not telling me to just make the pain go away, are you?" he mildly notes. "And I don't think you're telling me a story about cancer and the trauma of mortality, either."

He's heard that correctly; I'm smiling when I shake my head.

———

I've brought my list of demands. No echoing and mirroring please. If I announce,

> I find no peace, and all my war is done,
> I fear and hope, I burn and freeze like ice,

I don't want him to respond as all my grad school shrinks used to, *I think I'm hearing some ambivalence in what you say.*

He nods. But, "Did I just do that to you?"

"Hm, I thought you were asking something substantive, not just paraphrasing me for my own benefit. Asking is great, I like it—but when someone paraphrases in that routine way, I feel as though my own words are being set aside, disrespected."

"It's true, I *was* asking. Okay. I'll have to think a little more about it, but I expect I can probably agree to that one."

"Then, there's something about pleasure that might be important. I don't know how to say it properly: I've gotten hold of an intuition that if things can change for me, it won't be through a very grim process. It won't happen as I always used to imagine in the old days, by delivering myself up for good at the door of the Law. I used to take one deep masochistic breath, and determine I was ready to surrender to the disciplinary machine—in enough pain to have to do it—but then of course I didn't know how to, and couldn't sustain my resolve anyway; and nothing about the therapy would work. Now it seems that if anything can bring me through to real change, it may be only some kind of pleasure. Does this make any sense to you?"

"Oh, yeah, it makes plenty of sense. Let me think about how it feels to me to be doing this . . . No, grim truly isn't the feeling. At least it's never very grim for very long. I have to tell you it's often *painful*—"

My slightly secret smile. "I tolerate pain OK."

"But pleasure, yes, a fair amount of pleasure is what keeps me at it, too. Different kinds of. The people I take on as patients are people I anticipate liking and having some fun with. I could with you, I'm pretty sure. We'd invent our ways."

"Good. Then—well, I need you to be my age or older."

"Where does *that* come from?"

"I don't know, but something tells me I can't face learning after months of therapy that you're, like, thirty-two."

"No. I'm forty-eight. I think I can promise always to remain older than you."

"Also—these next ones are far more important—I've been a feminist for as long as I've known what the word means, and I need for my therapist to be one. I don't have a laundry list or a litmus test to define it, but I'm assuming you probably know if you are."

This gets two, near-expressionless nods.

"And—I guess I'm not asking you about your sexual orientation, but queer stuff is so central in my life. Even aside from my own sexuality, it's at the heart of just about everything I do and love as an adult. Also if the world is divided—and it seems to be, doesn't it?—between people who are inside the experience of the AIDS epidemic and people who are outside it, then I seem to be way inside.

"So probably if I'm going to relax with you at all, I need to start out knowing—as much as it's possible to know—that you aren't phobic about all that. Actually, that you feel very fine and at home about it."

—————

"I guess I'm not asking you about your sexual orientation," I said— and he nodded soberly. I don't know what I'm supposed to assume about this. The very emphatic recommendation of Shannon came from another shrink, one who knew me pretty well. And experience shows that I'm one of those people who when others say to me,

"I'm just sure you'd get
along marvelously with
X"—then X is gay.

But Shannon isn't immediately legible in this way. It's true, gratefully his hand is un-wedding-ringed, his desk undecked with any wife and kids. But couldn't that be from reticence or delicacy?

Still, if delicacy, that would itself please and suit me.

He doesn't *look* delicate. Or gay.

He looks more like a guy. Someone who's never viewed his body, or had or wanted it viewed, much as an object of desire. Someone also for whom, maybe—unlike me or most anyone I love—his entitlement to exist, the OK-ness of being who and as he is, has never seemed very seriously questionable.

It worries me: how could someone like that have learned to think or feel? Seemingly he's not even Jewish. I already know the demographics of people in the mental health field are even more mixed than their assumptions and training; I can't encounter only Viennese refugees, don't even want to. Still,

> this nasal-voiced, corn-
> fed Dutchman from the heartlands:
> has he any *soul*?

And he's saying, "I don't want to say, 'Some of my best friends are . . . '"

Then an ungirdled, self-satisfied laugh. Says he works a lot with lesbian and gay clients; also gives time to the Lesbian and Gay Health Project over on Ninth Street.

He adds, "But there's honestly no one template I want to get people to fit into. I'm certainly not in this profession because I want to turn out insurance salesmen." He produces the formulation confidently, as though he's said it with great success to a thousand previous patients. And there's an additional, habituated-sounding laugh that goes with its articulation.

"Or at least," he amends, "that's what I always used to say to people. Then one day I found myself saying it to a perfectly nice man who sold insurance. Maybe, really, that's fine too?" A chuckle.

It's a good thing Shannon is not trying to recruit me for Aetna or Allstate, because he'd have his work cut out for him.

At least, it's news to me if they're keen on hiring trousered, crewcut, 250-pound, shy middle-aged women writers, whether depressed or not, to promote financial instruments to American homeowners.

Moving toward the door of his office, we make a tentative appointment for the next week and agree that I'll call him if I decide I want to keep it. I say I expect I will—but of the four therapists I've arranged to "interview," there's one more I haven't seen, and it wouldn't do to prejudge. The fourth one's a psychiatrist; a possible advantage is that she could prescribe the antidepressants I'm also thinking of starting. All this makes sense to Shannon, and in mutual friendliness and uncertainty we part.

But oh my. Even stepping down to the waiting room, I think I feel it already, the uneven double pressure that will whirlpool around this decision.

From one direction come words, my scornful private words, the ones I never say, among the worst I know. Fatuous is one. Complacent another. Stupid is the overarching theme. "How dumb would someone have to be . . ." thrusts suddenly into my head— how dumb, specifically, to see me as someone likely to be charmed or reassured in this way?

Is Shannon stupid? In the abstract, I've wrapped my mind around the unlikeliness of connecting with a shrink who's brilliant or even an intellectual. I can even doubt that I'd choose to deal with one. But that's in the abstract; in the real world, stupidity isn't a lack but an aggressively positive, entitled presence, and to chafe my own mind and psyche raw against it would be cruel medicine.

These fiercely devaluing phrases:

a storm driving hail-
seeds and mica flakes of snow
against the deep hill.

For from the other side there come no words.

Does the defense rest?

Yes, there could have been words in thoughtful Shannon's favor: the quiet elegance of some of his answers, kindness of them all, attractive queer avoirdupois, the very evident readiness not only to respect but enjoy an idiom not his own. But what I find instead is only, wordlessly, this: a fact of life in its staggering specific gravity

> present to me, like
> earth, less as a new need than
> a new element.

If my heart held an image then, perhaps it came from the *Scientific American* of my early teens. Do I remember or imagine it? An article about Harry Harlow's baby monkey studies, we'll say. Painfully flashbulbed black-and-white photos, plus drawings in the gently stippled, tactile style of the magazine, show hairy infants cowering in avoidance of their wire experimental "mother," rigged though she is to yield milk if only they'd give her spiky frame a nuzzle. They won't. Where they cling instead is to the milkless, white puffy breast of her sister, also wire, but padded with cathectible terrycloth that dimples with their embrace . . .

Who would dare try to break back from the terrycloth bosom, one by one, those scrawny, holding, ravenous, loving toes?

Then let the same fearless person try to come between me and my appointment next week with the peony sunlight of this office, airy rondure into whose

> yielding lap I seem
> already to have leapt for
> good. The oddest thing!

When I called to say yes

> . . . can I even swear
> he didn't say, "Oh goody"?
>   Hold the date—I'm *there*.

2

It's hard, this part. In the new diaries I'd undertake for the first few days of every January when I was a kid, I'd shipwreck on the need to introduce all the *dramatis personae* at once. My older sister Nina was good at that, though. So this is from her 1958 diary: "I'm an 11-year-old girl called Nina Kosofsky. I weigh 75 lbs., and I have dark hair and dark eyes. Quite

> often I am a
> bit short-tempered. Yours truly
> enjoys reading, dolls,

dancing, writing stories, poems, and plays. Hiking is also in my line.

"Buttons is our almost-7-year-old cat. She is very fat and everyone always thinks that she is about to have kittens. (She can't, though, she's been spade.) She is very unfriendly with other cats of both sexes. She is all black, gray, and white striped, except for her orangey stomach.

"David is my 4- going on 5-year-old brother. He looks quite a lot like me. David is very cute when he wants to be (and that's almost always), and he knows it. He doesn't talk babytalk or lisp, except that he sometimes changes j's to d's and th's to v's.

"Mommy.

My mother's name is
Rita Goldstein Kosofsky,
and she's 36.

She also looks a lot like me. Mommy is *very* even-tempered. Unlike a lot of mothers, she (almost) always likes, and usually uses, new ideas. I love her very, very much.

"Daddy. Leon J. Kosofsky, my father, is 38 years old. He is not fat, but just big. He is mostly bald except for some hair around the edges of his head. He is sometimes

rather short-tempered
which I think is my fault, but
usually he

is *very* kind and understanding. Daddy can sometimes look almost exactly like Yul Brynner. I love him very much.

"Eve, my sister, is 8 years old. She has light hair and freckles. She is *really* a 'book-worm.' I guess that that must be part of the reason for her being old for her age. Eve is quite plump (she outweighs me by 4 lbs.). I

seem to remember
her being even-tempered,
more when she was young,

although she is still very easy-going."

In fact it comes readily enough, the task of scene-setting. There's no pleasure to me at this point, only dread, in invoking a Kosofsky world in this or any space. But I discover that to tell something *to Shannon*— in fact, to tell anything to Shannon— makes a wholly new motive I all but shamelessly indulge.

No, the harder part is in telling it now; choosing now to thread the
viscera of the labyrinth of

> what I didn't know
> and when I didn't know it,
> and what *that* felt like,

not to know things; I don't even mean big things, but the most ordinary ones.

"The canonical areas, love and work—those are weirdly good for me.
I mean, of course there are problems, some big ones, but it doesn't
seem as though those areas are where The Problem lives. Assuming
there is such a thing as The Problem."

"'The Problem' . . . ?"

"Oh, I guess . . . the ontological problem. What's the Matter with
Eve." Why she and life seem to refuse each other. Because after all

> it isn't that things
> for me don't *work*. They do! They
> do, in many ways,
>
> so beautifully:
> if anything, *that* scares me
> because if things change

(and I need them to change), wouldn't it likely be for the worse?

I expect there are tears here. Not copious tears, but seeping ones:
I think of them contemptuously as the tears of privilege.

"It's frightening to feel so little attachment to a life that's so full of
the things other people long for—rightly long for, I think: a lot of intimacy, enough money, peace and privacy, intellectual stimulation,
plenty of recognition, time for my own work, no violence, both par-

ents living, mostly good health, a long, tender relationship with my fella, oodles of terrific friends . . . It's not that these things don't seem miraculous. They do: when I was a kid I certainly didn't expect to have most of them. It almost seems miraculous, being a woman, just never to have been raped or battered or had an unwanted pregnancy. I've the most acute sense that things not only could be infinitely worse, but actually are for most people. Though I can't imagine why that's supposed to be a cheering realization!

"But somehow the goodness of these good things doesn't find its way inside me. I go after them purposefully enough, but when they arrive it's as if I didn't know how to reach my hand out and pull them in."

There's a Christian hymn with lines I'm fond of,

> For the beauty of the earth,
> For the beauty of the skies,
> For the love that from our birth
> Over and around us lies

—maybe perversely fond of, because what I like them for is the pathos of how the beauty and love are described as being everywhere in the world but inside us.

> I *was* a morbid,
> sentimental kid, I'm sure
> of that, and the thought
>
> of dying young was
> a good friend to me often.
> Sure it sounds funny,
>
> but to think of death
> brought me a sense of safety.
> Rest. Of being held.

"Another form it maybe took, though, is that I never, ever wanted to have children of my own."

"Do you have any?"

"No! Never *have* wanted. The friends who've known me longest say it was always true. What I mostly can remember about that is a long, bottomless draught of reproach against my parents for having made me be born. And, oh, I remember thinking—thinking it in so many words, maybe I was eight, maybe eleven—'I could never stand for *any*one, for any

child I had borne, to
feel this unanswerable
reproach against *me.* ' "

TALKING ABOUT HER WISH TO DIE OR NO LONGER BE, OCCASIONED BY HER
FINDING A LUMP ON HER NECK WHICH IMMEDIATELY HAS HER THINKING
ABOUT CANCER. SHE TOLD ONLY HUSBAND AND ONE FRIEND. WHAT SHE DOES
NOT TELL IS HER EXCITEMENT AT THE POSSIBILITY OF CANCER AND DYING,
WHICH SHE NURSES AND WHICH HAS NUMEROUS FACETS—GUILT OVER A
"WICKED" THOUGHT, SOME RELIEF, SOME ANXIETY, ETC. WHAT STRIKES ME IS
THE PASSIVITY AND THE SENSE OF BEING RESCUED BY DEATH. SHE RESONATES
TO THE RESCUE—BEING SWEPT OFF BY DEATH LIKE BEING TAKEN OFF BY SOME-
ONE ON A WHITE HORSE. MENTIONS ASSOCIATIONS OF LAWRENCE OF ARABIA, *AT
THE BACK OF THE NORTH WIND*—THE IMAGE IS ONE OF LOSS OF BOUNDARIES
AND A MERGING WITH SILENT FIGURE NOW MALE BUT MAYBE NOT ALWAYS. IT IS
IN CONTRAST TO THE IMAGE OF HAVING TO ESTABLISH HER SELF IN INTERAC-
TION W/ AN OTHER. THESE BOTH ARE DISTINCT FROM THE IMAGE OF A WARM,
LOVING, CARING RELATIONSHIP W/ FRIENDS—WHICH HOWEVER STILL SEEMS A
MATURE EVOLUTION OF THE RESCUE FANTASIES.

Shannon wants to know if I feel as if I don't really exist; or whether maybe I'm just pretending to exist; or if I feel as if I'm watching my life through someone else's eyes. But it isn't any of those failures. It's a different failure.

Do I feel like a fraud? No, not particularly. Oh, and have I ever been suicidal?

I know that I've never attempted suicide. So I guess I know by now I never would or could. Because there was that stretch of years—my teens, my twenties—when, hour after hour, the thought of it was constantly with me, and I gave myself many a fine old scare with it. No, I truly never even think about it now.

And why it never happened . . . Well, say that a suicide has to be several things at once:

a wish not to be,
an aggression against the
living, a message:

far as I can tell
I meant no message death had
words to deliver.

Meant no violence
to others' lives. Simply this.
The wish not to be.

———————

I arrive with photos for show-and-tell. Diffidently, but Shannon is game for them. Amazing the mix (I think now) of pride and peevishness behind my choice of these pictures! I was thinking, I guess, of therapy as the place for turning the old twining pains into grownup, full-throated grievances. But also want Shannon to see in us that same

unbroken circle
of the handsome, provincial
Jewish family

the photos all mean to offer evidence of. Want the taste in his mouth of Nina puffing at her recorder, slightly cross-eyed; her castanet gaze as the "Spanish dancer" in a ballet recital at Dayton School of Dance; clothes matching, three kids doing blunt-scissored arts and crafts around a table.

In a tiny living room, the loveseat where my father assembles many of these tableaux: an endless parade of identical-sister dresses for Nina and Evie. Also a chain of testimonials to literacy—Mommy reading to Nina, Nina reading to me, me (precocious) puzzling it out to myself. Nobody's bothering to document by the time David, here still a happy butterball, comes to the Word.

A subplot. From the wall above the loveseat gaze down an anxious succession of rabbinic, existentially miserable faces. The brushwork ranges from like-Cézanne to like-Rouault; they're from the Dayton Art Institute, the circulating collection, and they too have come far from Brooklyn.

We *are* good-looking.
All Mediterranean,
all with fine brown frames

and those sparkling or
soulful, extravagant-lashed
eyes of chocolate

—all but a dorkily fat, pink, boneless middle child; one of my worst nicknames is "Marshmallow."

It's true, it's hard to see my mother's eyes. Except in a couple of languid shots from her twenties, she suffers from "photo face," the painful, dissociated clamp-eyed rictus

tugging at the cords
of her neck to make her look
like Nancy Reagan

or a tiny Anne Sexton. Another result of this tension is that any child young enough to be held will be transfixed by the flashbulb at some precarious angle to her body, or seem to pop from her arms as toast from a toaster.

Shannon wonders at whom her photo face is aimed. I guess at my father, always behind the flash? But really, the audience for these photos is the four New York grandparents—especially her mother, Nanny, who sews all the dresses and will want to see (at least, will be supposed to want to see) how family-like they make the young family appear.

Nina, on the other hand, displays the googly eyes in their platonically ideal form, and at this moment of Western culture that makes her "look like Annette Funicello." Uncanny how frontal, as toddler and child, she always manages to be—whether in the mode of cute or seductive;

> there's something perfect
> about her, something that gives
> a snap to snapshots.

It's also clear she loves her baby sister, if awkwardly. Eyes glued to the camera, she holds on as if for life to my waist or leg—me apparently struggling to withdraw from the picture, from her attentions. In the pictures from Dayton, I'm never quite there. It's as though I might will my whole being into my fingertips, and from them into something else through touch—a stuffed panda, my other hand, a book or cat, the fabric of a skirt.

Now, in the fifteen or twenty years since she's vanished, I tell Shannon, I never think about my sister's eyes. (*Vanished,* he wants to know? Well, yes—from us. She won't have any contact with us other four: she, her three kids, her husband, somewhere in Georgia or South Carolina. The one time my parents turned up on her doorstep, she threatened to call the cops.) But sometimes, in a low-vamped flat pump like she wore in her teens, I'll see somebody's brown, dry, round little muffin of a foot, with the toe divisions sexily shadowed at the top, and I'll—well, I guess I'll think about that, some. But it's not that I can't bear her absence from my life. I don't really miss her, as it happens; she was so difficult.

That kind of thing is why I say I don't quite have emotions.

I haven't brought teenage pictures. Until one, stylized shot where I'm nineteen, eyes crinkled with laughter and embarrassment as Hal, who's twenty-three, is pushing a morsel of our wedding cake into my mouth. Empathetically, urgingly, his mouth gapes toward mine like a mother bird's.

> "Is there *any* way
> this Hal can be sweet as he
> looks?" Yeah. And then some,

as seen a few years later in the small circle of unspeakably tender, slightly sad protection he creates for me in a visit to my parents' house. Those are years of acute depression for me, the years that convince me I can't bear to bring my mind close again to the Kosofsky world.

For that matter, the aegis of Hal's sweetness isn't so different from what was shed by my large, brooding-jawed father in the few Dayton photos where he comes out from behind the camera. Unlike Hal's, his sweetness is generalized by shyness. It seldom condenses around one person, unless my mother; almost unseen but content, Evie when she can will only grasp his finger, hold tight to the crease of his baggy trousers—who wouldn't?

Recent pictures—professional ones, this time—are from my folks' fiftieth anniversary. Mother sends Daddy her brutal photo face. Her real face, which turns out to be inquisitive, mischievous, and longing, gravitates helplessly (though she isn't trying to help it) toward the un-made-up, white-framed, down-to-earth visage of W.—the new, cherished intimate, a slightly older, German-Jewish photographer and professional woman whose gravely literal aura and round eyes are not so unlike my dad's.

My own eyes, blue with the electric blue of my shirt, are also magnetized: blotting up as if passively, one by one, each of the three.

———————

"Yes, we always used
to joke at home about my
mom being a dyke."

"What do you mean, '*joke*'? For that matter, what do you mean 'always'?"

"Well, as long as I can remember, at least from my teens, it was this family . . . joke. Not that it was treated as something that could really happen. But as a true fact about how my mother *was*, what interested her—sure."

"Like what? How would it sound?"

"*You* sound as if you haven't heard this particular family joke before."

"No, I haven't. Though I might like to! I get the feeling it's very Kosofsky?"

"Yeah, that's true—one of those things that make a girl proud to be a Kosofsky."

"Were they mean jokes? Would she make them herself?"

"I don't think they were mean at all. Like, she would come back from swimming at the Y, and there'd be a lot of joking about her hanging around the locker room to ogle naked women."

"And she would say it too?"

"Oh, yeah, of course, it was her own account. Or she would joke about crushes she used to have on her teachers, or on women athletes when she was a kid. I think I heard a lot more about Babe Didrickson than most English teachers' daughters do."

"Was there ever serious talk, or just these jokes?

"Only the jokes. I promise you, that was how we dealt with every-thing sexual. At least—until she was almost seventy, and met W."

"Tell me some more of them."

"Oh, it's hard for me to remember. There was a standing routine about how she always wanted her hair shorter, how she could never get her haircutters to believe how short she really wanted it. Then as soon as my father or someone would say her hair looked nice, she'd say it was time for a new haircut."

"But in these pictures she doesn't look mannish, does she?"

"No! She's dainty, dainty."

———

"The best thing," I'm telling Shannon one day, "I think the thing I'd most want somebody to know about how I've lived . . . Oh, I do seem to be confessing to you that I

> have the secret vice
> of mentally writing my
> obituary!

Do you think you can bear it?"

Shannon mimes invitation.

"What I'm proudest of, I guess, is having a life where work and love are impossible to tell apart. Most of my academic work is about gay men, so it might seem strange to you that I would say that—not being a man, not even, I don't think, being gay. But it's still true. The work is *about* sex and love and desire, to begin with—like your work I sup-pose—so it's almost bound to be involving at that intimate level. But beyond that, even—Oh, where to start!

"Well, I should say that one true thing about me is that my love is *with* gay men."

I don't quite understand what the term "fag hag" means. Anyway, I don't understand what it could mean nowadays. "Fag hag" conjures

up for me a scene at a bar in the 1950s where a lot of self-hating people are getting very drunk—me, I don't even drink.

Anyway, sometimes I think the term "fag hag" has a fake specificity. Maybe it does the same work that, say, "nigger lover" did in the
'50s and '60s: to punish anyone who just doesn't feel some form of
contempt that their society says they ought to feel. So I don't have any
sense whether or not the term describes me. And of course "It isn't
that I like or love all gay men—naturally I don't. I love the particular
people I do love.

"Still . . . still . . . all these aspects of my life are so intimately involved with each other."

"Could you give me a for-instance?"

"Well, okay, I'll tell you about Michael. Michael Moon. He's the person I'm living with now."

"He's the 'fella' you mentioned a while ago?"

"No, no! Hal is my fella—Hal's still my fella. But he teaches in New
York, so we only see each other on weekends—we've been doing that
for decades now. No,

> he's not Michael Moon,
> Michael's a gay man with a
> fella of his own,

and I guess you'd call our relationship 'best friends.' But that's wrong,
I don't know a category that describes my friendship with Michael."
There'd be nothing untrue about saying I'm in love with him. Our
bond is very passionate, at least for me; it preoccupies me a lot; it's
very physical, though we don't have sex; and I guess the emotional
weather of my day will most often be determined by Michael's emotional weather.

"So what comes to you in this relationship?"

"Gee, it's changed me in a hundred big and little ways. There's so
much pleasure! I've always had a lot of funniness in my life, even
when I was near-suicidal, but before Michael I don't think I knew any-

one who could *always* make me laugh out loud, laugh with my whole
body, anytime it occurred to them to want to. Not sure I even knew
what the feeling was like before.

> No, Michael has these
> big, queer, expressive talents—
> ventriloquism,
>
> esoterica,
> tells stories so they stay told;
> his people seem more
>
> real than real people.
> I never feel as if I've
> read a book until
>
> Michael has channeled
> it for me—really, that goes
> for my own life too.

And what's rarest is how he uses these things to make a world, a kind
of warm, musical, hilarious private culture to share with the people he
loves.

"But then that goes with being a complicated, saturnine guy. He
came out late, finished college late, started his career late—there are
places in his life that are still raw with abjection and anger. Which is
almost impossible for me to bear."

I'm very addicted to Michael's sunshine. I often think I'd do anything to obtain or keep it.

Shannon wants to know if I have other friendships that work at all
this way. The weird thing is that I do: I've moved from job to job so often as an academic, and the map is spangled with friends I've been in
love with rather like this. By now I feel almost promiscuously skilled
in such intimacy.

"A funny fate for someone who's so shy—as though, if you don't have the talent to fake intimacy a lot of the time, you're *forced* to do the real thing?"

————————

I ASKED HER TO TALK SOME ABOUT HOW BEING IN HER FAMILY WAS FOR THE VARIOUS MEMBERS.

————————

My mother, my mother, my mother, my mother, my mother!

"Y-e-eah? Something you wanted to tell me about your mom?"

"Oh, my mom! You know, I refer to her as 'my mom,' but not even that is exactly true.

"We never called her Mom. She would have hated it. I only use the word now, when I mention her to other people, to try and sound more normal. My brother still won't use it."

"Why did she hate it?"

"American? Slangy? Uncultured? I don't know, but she did. She and my father had this ideal of the 'Old World family'—where children were still childlike, and, oh, I'm not sure, everyone played piano sonatas together."

"So what did you call her?"

"Mommy."

"And then when you got older?"

"Mommy!"

"Really?"

"Well, no, *I* don't. It sounds way too abject. I never do now. But I did till I went away to college. It's always seemed as though the only alternative was 'Mother,'

but that's so much too
stiff and frigid."

        "So what *do*
you call her?"

            "Mother."

————

WE TALKED MOSTLY ABOUT HER FATHER. HE APPEARS TO HAVE BEEN CON-
STANTLY INVOLVED WITH GATHERING INFORMATION FOR NO OBVIOUS END. HE
HAS CONTINUED TO TAKE A COURSE A SEMESTER TO THIS DAY IN ALMOST ANY
AND EVERY SUBJECT AREA. E WAS VERY AFRAID OF HIM BUT IS NOT SURE WHY
OTHER THAN REMEMBERING HOW HE WOULD GET ANGRY—PUFFING UP AND
TURNING RED—AS IF ABOUT TO EXPLODE—BUT NOT PHYSICALLY VIOLENT.
MORE TO HER FEAR THAN SHE CAN ACCESS AT PRESENT. LIKE E HE IS SHY. SHE
ENDS SAYING SHE IS GLAD TO BE TALKING ABOUT HER FATHER BUT ISN'T SURE
WHY.

————

MORE DESCRIPTION OF FATHER TO ME BUT I HAVE A HARD TIME GETTING A CO-
HESIVE PICTURE OF HIM, ONE THAT DOESN'T FEEL FRAGMENTED TO ME. I'M
NOT SURE HOW TO VIEW THIS DIFFICULTY I'M HAVING. FATHER SEEMS VITAL
AND ALIVE, NOT ESPECIALLY DEPRESSED OR DISAPPOINTED, BUT SOMEWHAT
ALIEN TO E. POSSIBLY HIS INNER LIFE JUST IS VERY FRAGMENTED OR OTHER-
WISE SOMEHOW INGENUOUS. ALSO THERE ARE THE ANGER EPISODES AND HER
FEAR OF HIM. FEAR OF HIM ALWAYS (FROM CHILDHOOD) TIED TO FEAR FOR
HIM—WILL HE EXPLODE, E.G. HAVE HEART ATTACK? YET E NEVER DOUBTED HE
LOVED ALL THREE CHILDREN—STEADY AFFECTION DIFFERENT FROM MOTHER.
E'S BROTHER EXPERIENCED HIM AS KIND "GENTLE GIANT" AND APPRECIATED
ALL THE KNOWLEDGE. BUT THERE IS THE FACT THAT E HAS CONSIDERABLE
MATH DIFFICULTY WHICH SHE TRACES BACK TO HIS TRYING TO TEACH HER
MATH CONCEPTS. ALSO ASSOCIATES HER POOR MEMORY, "ALLERGY TO INFORMA-
TION," WITH HIS BEING MR. INFORMATION. I ON THE OTHER HAND EXPERI-
ENCE HER AS PLENTY CURIOUS, WELL INFORMED??

————

SENSE OF MOTHER AS WISHFUL, "INVENTIVE" VIS-À-VIS REALITY. DID I TELL YOU
ABOUT MY MOTHER EXPLAINING WHAT TO DO IF YOU GOT LOST IN A STORE—
TOLD ME TO ASK SOMEONE TO TAKE ME TO THE LOST AND FOUND AND WAIT
THERE FOR HER. I VISUALIZED A MEZZANINE WITH A NUMBER OF CHILDREN

SIPPING SODAS AND WAITING. LATER I GOT LOST IN DEPT. STORE, COULDN'T
FIND MOTHER—WENT TO SALESPERSON AND ASKED TO BE TAKEN TO LOST AND
FOUND—THEY COULDN'T FIGURE OUT WHAT I MEANT, EXPLAINED THAT LOST
AND FOUND WAS A DRAWER WITH LEFT-BEHIND GLASSES AND GLOVES IN IT—
FRIGHTENED AND IN THE WRONG. ANOTHER TIME E WAS LEFT TO TAKE BUS
HOME WITHOUT MUCH MONEY, "THAT'S OKAY, THE BUSES HAVE A SPECIAL FARE
FOR CHILDREN"—NOT SO. MOM'S PLEASURE, PRIDE IN INVENTIVENESS AND
NOT BEING "LITERAL-MINDED," VIS-À-VIS FATHER AS PEDANTIC, LITERAL-
MINDED.

———————

Years ago, David sent me a great analysis of certain pivotal moments
in both our adult lives, moments he labeled

"acknowledging the
reality of." Of, like,
poverty. Weather.

Death, or pain, or systemic injustice. Or that certain processes take ac-
tual time.
All the things we'd learned to be so proud of magicking away, as
kids—waving the Rita-conferred wand of "ambiguity," imagination.
Not for us those plodding dualisms, the ones less agile people got
stuck in like dinosaurs in the tar pits.
No original sin. None of the immemorial quarrels into which peo-
ple are drafted long before their birth.
"For sure, it gives a freshness to our adult encounters!"
The freshness of slow learners . . .

———————

Vocabulary
list: Nuance. Ambivalence.
Gamine. Wistful. Brisk.

"I think I had three distinct modes of being, as a kid.

"One, I could disappear from view—worst fear, and great protection, of the middle child.

"Two, I could be a caretaker.

"Or three, I could actively threaten my parents, frighten them, make them even more anxious and defensive than, I now see, they must have felt from day to day.

"I *was* awfully competitive. I'm sure I must have lodged pretty deeply under my mother's skin."

This seems to surprise Shannon. Also interest him; but he says, "This is one I'll need some convincing on. Because I don't know how to take it for granted that a child can be that threatening to a grownup.

"I think about relating to my kids—I've felt a lot of things, but threatened, no, challenged in that particular way—no, I don't think I've felt that; I don't think someone would necessarily feel that."

Well, of course, I say,

you're a hell of a
lot better analyzed than
we Kosofskys were!

When I tell Hal about Shannon's skepticism,

he laughs and laughs and
laughs. I have to hammer him
on the back to stop.

He's known me from almost back then—a girl with long red hair pulled behind a blue ribbon—and he takes the uncanniness quite for granted.

I'm thinking how much the spookiness of that kid must have dwelt in the mix of fierce verbal aptitude with the already raging depression. Almost-constant efforts to deprecate or blunt the force of both of those must have made her all the creepier. (At least to anybody tuned in on those wavelengths.)

That Rita could tune in on them I'm certain.

We're on precocity, its queerness, its sinister ramifications. Shannon says, with his candor, "I'm just trying to think how things could have happened differently, even around a child who was the way you describe yourself. I guess the way I'm thinking of it is, there has to be an important set of ways in which, after all, this *is* still a *kid*. And likes kid things, and has kid needs . . ."

"Yes," I say, with a complicated bitterness, "I was extremely aware of that. I hated it! It seemed like a humiliating joke."

"But," he goes on, "now I'm imagining how I would treat someone like that if I'd been one of your parents. I'm thinking there's this part of you that's a child, that I would want to, you know—tend, and nourish"—he makes a stroking motion here of one hand with the other—"and play with. And then there's this other part that's so bright—and that would be loads of fun too. There's all the encouragement to give, and the, I don't know, the chemistry sets to play with or ballet barres to set up."

Yes, I say, we got plenty of that kind of encouragement.

"But," I also enunciate, "what you completely do not seem to catch on to about these two parts of the kid is that they are *not separate*. They are constantly whirlpooling around in each other—and the basic rule is this: that each one has the power to poison the other one. So what being a kid was like for me was, at the same time, like being an adult in bad drag as a child, and being a child in bad drag as an adult." I *was* abject, incompetent, and powerless. (Me weeping copiously all this time; expressing myself forcefully all the same.)

I'm angry at having to say all this to Shannon. I'm angry and frightened at the ingenuousness of the formulation he's offered. Though he didn't say so, I feel sure it was a description of the family he grew up in—and their invocation sends me reeling between contempt and envy.

But, funnily, I seem actually to have given him some pause. "I think I am finally really hearing this," he says."I need to get more from you about it, but I think I am starting to be able to imagine it.

"It's just so much easier for me to envision things in discrete parts. But then you come along and smudge up the barriers, and it's really different. It's important for you to keep doing that—I really think I am getting it."

Deconstruction 101, I do *not* say impatiently.

Then he asks, when I was involved in these scouring devaluations of myself, could I tell whose voice it was that I was hearing in my head?

Me: "I think that's an important question"—meaning I can't answer it—"but there's something else I want to say about it. One of the big features of being this kind of kid is that you articulate quite an elaborate inner space, full of all kinds of voices. Not to say the voices don't come from anywhere, they do—but they don't come *directly* from anywhere. There's a lot of time and echoey, experimental space for them to take on a life of their own. There are all the fearful—and worse, hopeful—gaps between what you'd want to say and what you can (as a kid) manage to say. There's the insuperable problem of *as whom* or as what one can say anything—well, there's lots of room inside for the echoes of all these voices that don't seem to be going anywhere else."

So, you mean, he asks, you would be thinking one thing, but then you would say to yourself, "Nobody's going to do what I want them to unless I act like a kid"?

Oh, no, it's worse than that. I don't believe I was ever, ever cynical. I expect it would have been much easier if I had been. I could *know*, but I couldn't *say to myself*, that I would have to do something-or-other in the persona "kid."

"So it was as if I were a method actor: it was my job to propel my-self into 'kid' by the very force of my sincerity, I would have to *want to* be 'kid.' But for the same reason I wasn't very good at it—my child-likeness was always too much, too insistent, or off in some way or an-other. And because of this, of course, I could never be anything like centered; I just got so, so flung around. My being was always hollow-ing out, or whirlpooling, or flooding. I don't think I was vindictive, I mean, but everything I did or felt had to be 'with a vengeance.' There wasn't any mode of being that didn't feel entirely spoiled by all the falseness."

I guess I've been staring off at the grim distance as I produce this account. Because when I turn back toward Shannon at the end of it, looking for the impassively friendly countenance that always greets me, what I find is—his face buried in one hand, head shaking back and forth in some weird combination of mock despair and real de-spair and disbelief.

I'm still not quite sure why.

But it's kind of a powerful thing.

"You were a mess!" is all he at first manages to say. "A mess! I hear it!

"It's that the you I see when I look at you, sitting there on the couch so nicely, is the product of an arduous and almost endless labor. You really were very, very different from the way you are now—the person I know is someone who's been torturously polished, rubbed,

shaped, repainted, pinked,
molded . . . You've done so much!
                                You're
really different."

———

TALKS ABOUT THE FEELING OF BEING RESPONSIBLE FOR ME —FOR MY IN-
VOLVEMENT, FOR DRAWING OUT MY BEST INTEREST AND INTELLIGENCE TO IN-
TERACT WITH HER. LIKENS IT TO TRYING TO ENGAGE HER MOTHER WHO WOULD

INTERACT WITH HER AS A PERSON, AS IF ADULT FOR A TIME AND THEN ARBI-
TRARILY CUT THAT OFF AND TREAT HER LIKE A CHILD BUT IN AN INAUTHENTIC
WAY. "NURSERY SCHOOL TEACHER'S VOICE," SINGSONG, OVERENUNCIATED,
SACCHARINE.

> —some estranging sense,
> radiating discomfort,
> of "mother" with "child."
>
> Hating that: my first
> memory of real hatred.
> A blade. A glass wall.

Did she teach nursery school?

"Yeah, for a while—teaching half days when I was seven or eight, at a Jewish nursery school.

"But it wasn't a big success. She wound up hospitalized with a bleeding ulcer. It was actually very scary."

"The teaching caused that? It must have been a handful, with the three of you–your brother was, what, five?"

"All I know is the family legend about it. Come to think of it, there were two legends about her ulcer. Both of them naming women as the cause, as a matter of fact.

"One of them ran the nursery school—an Orthodox woman who somehow, inadvertently, I guess ground my mother's gut into powder with some mix of perfectionism, disorganization, and passive aggression. I don't remember her well, but even at eight, I thought I could see how she'd have that effect.

"Then there was this other legend, about my best friend's mother. She wasn't involved with the school, but I think she must've been another grating superego for my mother. She was bigger, louder, more confident, more savvy—looking back, they must have been richer, too—and she would garden and sew and radiated briskness and *com-*

petence. The sewing was worst, because Nanny was a demon at sewing, and my mother didn't take to it at all. She and Jane came up with some project of making clown costumes for us that Halloween. That was the other thing that was supposed to have precipitated this ulcer."

"So she was a failure at working *and* at mothering."

"That must have been the message. It does sound awful."

But a few years later, a better-fated vocation: teaching high school English. It was so obvious that she was a terrific teacher—and she seemed so fond of her students. We pretended to be jealous of them, but David and I, at least, must have been proud of her, too. At least we're both teaching English today.

"And she?"

"Oh, she is too! Since they retired, she and my father are immersed in this world of teaching and learning. 'Improving their minds.' Reading groups are the basic unit, I guess—she's always leading at least one—and they're in other groups that don't have a leader, and she teaches adult education courses, and they *take* courses, and then they do Elderhostels, and . . . It's pretty amazing. She's really valued. She's really good at it.

"And a funny thing is that they've lived in the same place all these years, so whenever I go anywhere with her, about half the people we see have been her students at one time or another—when they were three, or seventeen, or eighty-five, or some combination. They all express so much gratitude and admiration."

Shannon's wondering
how it all strikes me. And I'm
just shaking my head.

No simple way at
all. I used to have so much
contempt for middle-

brow culture, but hers
isn't that, it's real as real—
I've run out of ways

to devalue it
or set mine apart from it
—except for being

so hot to produce,
so impatient with being
a consumer of

all this shared culture.
It *does* seem utopian.
We do share all kinds

of values, the dream
of being surrounded by
students who are friends

and vice versa
and making space happen for
intimate reading

pleasure within that
grim surround of public lives
and *ressentiment*—

DESPITE TENSIONS BETWEEN THEM, USUALLY SPEAKS OF MOTHER AND FATHER
AS MONOLITH, "MY FOLKS" (ALMOST ALWAYS REALLY = MOTHER). BEEN THINK-
ING MAYBE WE SHOULD BE TALKING ABOUT A PARENTAL UNIT RATHER THAN A
MOTHER AND A FATHER, BUT I DON'T WANT TO GIVE UP ON FATHER—SOMEONE
WHO COULD PUNISH BUT DOESN'T, OR WHOM YOU CAN RELATE TO SO THAT HE
WON'T—SOMEONE WHO PROVIDES (NOT JUST MATERIALLY), PROTECTS AS WELL.

"I'm wondering if you were a holy terror," Shannon says one day. "In
certain ways you sound like what parents would perceive as quite a dif-

ficult kid. But also some, you sound malleable and passive. Do you have a sense of whether you seemed to your folks like a *good* child?"

"Oh, I hope so!" I'm fervent. "That was absolutely all I wanted to be."

"It *was?*"

"Oh, yeah. Is that queer? I literally can't remember a single time I deliberately made mischief. It's funny, I know I must have been a smart, creative kid—it must have been in my nature somewhere to be active, aggressive, even sadistic." The only actual motives I remember having, though, were almost abject. I'd have done anything on earth to win my parents' love and admiration, and keep far away from trouble.

"—oh, and I guess to keep *everyone* away from trouble. Like when my older sister got to be a teenager, she had fights with my parents that felt, to me, world-threatening. I was so timid, it seems to me, but I couldn't stop go-betweening. Go be a middle child, huh?"

"Oh, right, there you were in the middle."

"Yes, exactly—three years on either side. It *is* true, isn't it?—that birth order stuff makes a huge difference?"

"I'm never quite sure. It's not like I'm making controlled experiments, you know? But it felt like that to you?"

"Oh, it utterly did,

as if 'middle child'
were like an identity—
or the lack of one,

since it seemed the very essence of middle-childness to identify with everyone *but* myself." I remember, in fourth grade, reporting in show-and-tell on my sister's arithmetic homework.

"Oh, *that* syndrome—I think I do know that one," says Shannon, and narrates a *Twilight Zone* plot to illustrate—

But no, I never saw it. I'm thinking of a girl text: *Little Women*. (This, Shannon hasn't read.) Where the sister I yearned toward was not Jo the bookish butch, not pretty artistic Amy, nor—well, did anyone ever identify with Meg?—but rather

slow musical Beth,
called by her father "Little
Tranquility," whose

death in late girlhood
sets a seal of peace on her
stormy family.

"Birds in their little
nests agree"'s her favorite
song—even back then

I wondered, reading,
whether she was mentally
retarded or just

stimulus-averse
like me. But oh, the quiet
around such deathbeds!

How low the price of
love: just that one sister, so
willing, disappear.

WHY NOT COUNSELING FOR E'S EARLY DEPRESSION? PARENTS NOT INVOLVED IN
"THERAPY CULTURE"; IT IS FOR VERY SICK PEOPLE OR UNUSUAL CIRCUMSTANCES
(E.G., CHILD IN NEIGHBORHOOD WHO WAS EXPOSED TO EXHIBITIONIST). ALSO,
SENSE THAT THERAPISTS WILL INEVITABLY AND UNFAIRLY JUDGE AND CONDEMN
PARENTS. EARLY JOKES "SOMEDAY YOU'LL TELL SHRINK ON US," ALSO JOKES
ABOUT CHILDREN REPORTING PARENTS TO SPCC. E SAYS SHE STILL SHARES THESE
ATTITUDES SOME: CAUGHT IN DYNAMIC OF ACCUSATION-PROTECTIVENESS OF
PARENTS; ALSO WORRIES, IS SHE BADLY OFF ENOUGH TO MERIT HELP.

One day I pluck up courage to ask Shannon what he thinks of the way I tell these stories.

"I'm not sure yet what to think," he says."I was trying to describe the effect to myself this weekend as I was thinking about you"

(—ontological
net that transfigures me: I
exist on weekends?)

"Lots of the things you say make my blood run a bit cold—I think that happens at the places you mean it to happen. You're a good narrator, real vivid, obviously really bright in a pleasurable way."

Ah, "really bright." It reminds me of how many things about my life are, in Shannon's mild judgment, "nice."

"But there's something that puzzles me, too, in the way you tell these things. I'm sure it will make more sense to me soon, but now it doesn't. The way people in my business think about psychological development is crude, but we're used to assuming that there are certain, pretty usual and reliable indices of damage in how someone's personality is put together. There are a bunch of them, and certainly depression is tied in with several. But some important ones are things like—an intolerance of ambiguity. Or the lack of an ability to empathize."

I'm laughing. "I think I can see where you've got a problem on your hands."

"Well, yes! Because the amount of just plain unhappiness you've been describing seems to come in at an unexpected angle to—"

"Oh, I think I know. To a competence I have in saying it. Including the interpersonal competence, I guess. And my *total* tropism toward ambiguities. And even empathy."

"Mm-hmm. That's kind of what it sounds like so far."

A long, long silence
ensues. I'm struggling. Till I
ask in a new voice,

"Did you know how awful it would make me feel, for you to say that?"

It's the first time I've had the presence of mind to proffer a real-time report of so sudden a sinking feeling.

And for the very first time, I see Shannon make a commiserating face. I don't like it a bit—it's a face you'd make to coax a two-year-old out of a tantrum. But he only says, "Did it? I'm sorry. No, I didn't know it would. Can you tell why?"

It seems to me the reason is humiliatingly obvious. But I understand

if I can't kick this
door open, there isn't hope—
I kick it open.

"I feel as though you think I'm malingering."

"You do?"

His look shows surprise and curiosity.

"It's interesting you'd feel that. But no, that wasn't something I was thinking. Generally, it's not one of the first ten hypotheses liable to leap to mind when I don't understand something. About you, moreover, I really don't think that."

"Really?"

"Oh, really. Why is it in your mind, do you think? You're really worried that you're malingering?"

"Certainly! You really aren't?"

Shannon shakes his head slowly."I'm not even sure what it would mean to. Though I guess it could make sense in the context of someone who felt as if getting cancer was like winning a lottery."

Well, *yeah*. I'm nodding fervently. Won't he see it? "It's funny," I say, "I've been trying real hard to be truthful with you—I'm generally truthful, but especially with you. And yet there's something irreducible, so far, about my sense of not having a right to make this claim on your attention—not unless I can come up with something spectacular in the way of damage. Which sounds more and more unlikely. And it seems that must really skew our conversations."

Shannon's reflective. "This isn't the main question I want to ask about what you're saying," he says, "but just for the moment: I'm supposed to hear in it that you're liking to have my attention?"

I stare at him. Softly, "I'm loving it."

"You know, I feel quite unproblematical about giving you this attention—about your ability to make use of me."

"You do, for sure?"

"Mm. A very relaxing feeling for me. Well, relaxing in the sense that when it comes to (what we call) 'working hard,' I really do think I see what makes sense and how we can do it."

Pleasurably I
muse on "Oh, what you call 'what
we call "working hard"' . . ."

3

Of course I know dreams are a part of the process, and yet for ages—
no dreams. Then one day I arrive with this one to tell.

"Okay, I was in bed with my father—don't ask me how. He turned
to me and said, 'It drives me crazy

> to just turn over
> and go right to sleep with no
> sex. Let's have some sex!'

I'm unenthusiastic but I say, 'Well, okay, sure . . .' Then he gets up to
go pee or something. When he comes back into the room, I say, 'I've
been thinking about it, and I really don't want to. What would I tell my
shrink? There are a million things I still have to narrate to Shannon,
but if I had sex with my father, then we wouldn't get to talk about anything else for just months and months.'"

I know this silence—of mine, of Shannon's—from my creative writing classes. Where someone reads a piece, and there's the fraught
pause, its length increasingly comic and suffused, which I'll let go on
and on until eventually I'll murmur

"What's this piece doing?"
or even, "What does it know?"
    What does my dream know?

It seems likely to me that what it knows best is how to make me happy,

and give me as well
a succulent mouse to lay
at my master's door.

"But it's true, you know, it's so hard for me to talk with you about sex at all."

"Yeah, I guess." I would not say that eagerness characterizes his tone. At all. He says as if approvingly, "A lot of people I see never do get around to talking about it. Even after a long time. Somehow we'll talk about their jobs, relationships, crises, parents and children, without . . ."

"Really? Most people don't talk about sex?"

He shakes his head empirically.

"So you figure it's more my Freudian preconceptions—as a literary critic? I've certainly heard people say that critics use more Freud, and are more attached to concepts like libido, than actual psychologists are anymore."

"Nah, not really. I'm fairly interested in that stuff too. It's just that somehow it doesn't come up with that many people."

Oh, dear! my funny
valentine! fallen this flat—
I'm so mortified.

It worries me awfully, too, to find the threshold to sex-talk such a high one. I know I want to talk about sex; it's what I do for a living (the talking, I mean), and I'm good at that, used to it. But my own sexuality—do I even have one? It leaves me stony with puzzlement. I don't know what *it* is; neither do I know its relation to what *I* am.

Freud says somewhere that his patients learn not to mind language about sex because, first, his manner with them remains "dry" and, second, he convinces them it's inevitable anyway. I've always thought this passage sounds like a

> description of rape,
> of an unlubricated
> rape for that matter.

Yet, however fearfully, I've counted on these conditions to obtain in therapy (is it a rape fantasy?).

But Shannon has articulated no rule. Clearly not a rule that sex talk is inevitable. Any more than he's ever told me—what? that we can't touch, or I must say whatever's in my head.

This inexplicitness, it's one of the ways I'm slowly coming to think of him as "a bit of a slob." I'm embarrassed partly for him, convinced he's *doing this wrong.* Unspeakably anxious, as well, for myself, left all alone (it feels like) with way too much responsibility. How, in such loose-knit colloquy, to find a place for my desire? Or anger?

———

The next hour, heart thudding with determination, I hurl myself straight at it.

"So I want to try and enumerate to you some of the outlines of a sexuality. Is this OK with you?"

His nod; no more than that. Looking back, I like my courage here; I remember my long silence.

"Once a few years ago, writing the introduction to my first queer book, I thought maybe I ought to explain what my own sexuality was. But sitting down to it, all I could think of to say was, It's at all the far extremes. All the *contradictory* extremes."

Shannon's sober nod. I like it, but it's no help at this juncture.

"From one point of view, you'd have to say I'm incredibly unsexual, unexploratory. I've only had three sex partners in my entire life!

"And as far as 'having sex' goes, things couldn't possibly be more hygienic or routinized for me. When I do it, it's vanilla sex, on a weekly basis, in the missionary position, in daylight, immediately after a shower, with one person of the so-called opposite sex, to whom I've been legally married for almost a quarter of a century.

"I've learned to *like* it, you know, I have orgasms and it feels good, but it's not what I think of as sexual. It doesn't reverberate; it doesn't make a motive for me. It's as if that happens in one place; then in another place, feelings of really profound, even really body-centered love and tenderness for my partner; but I can't find any connection whatsoever between them.

"Does that"—I dig in my heels abruptly to demand—"make any sense to you?"

"I'm not sure yet," says
calm Shannon, "probably not.
Wait a while. It will.

Go on about all the contradictions, though."

"Okay, so here are these sex *acts*, totally isolated, going on for years and years. In that dimension I'm having sex, but I'm not sexual. At the same time, there's this very sexualizing *person* I am—whose work and politics and friendships, whose interpretive and teaching and lecturing life, talking and joking, reading, thinking, whatever, are probably as infused with sexual meanings and motives and connections—*gay ones*—as anybody's you're ever likely to meet.

"It's funny, in spite of how homely-looking I am and how shy, I think a fair number of people think of me as even an unusually sexy person. And it's not a facade, at all. The thinking, writing, talking, all the sociality and political struggle around sex: those are the most vibrant things in my life. It's just, they don't connect up genitally for me."

"They don't at all?"

"I think not, no. I can't think of any way in which they do."

"That's it, then? That's all
that goes on between you and
genitality?"

Well. No.

––––––––––

Since meanwhile—no, this isn't true anymore. But up until recently, from as far back into childhood as I can remember, I was somebody who, given the opportunity, would spend hours and hours a day in my bedroom masturbating. Really. Hours and hours.
"Well, don't most kids do that?"
Do most adults? I feel quickly foreclosed.
"What makes me remark on it, I guess, is that for me, that *is* what feels like sex. It's something that I could

yearn toward and be
lost in the atmosphere of.
To me, a whole world."

—And what, he wants to know, did that world feel like?
Which is the difficult thing.
There's a long pause.
"I'm going to say two things, and they aren't going to fit together, I see it now. That's all I can do.
"One of them is a description of

the aura of this
fantasy world. Warm. Golden.
Intoxicating.

Playful, too; attentive, deliciously attentive."

"And the other . . . ?"
"What's going on in these fantasies."

———————

Violence and pain.
Humiliation. Torture.
Rape, systematic.

I'm looking deliberately away from Shannon, toward the far corner of the room, as I say this, so I can't see his face. I wrench my eyes back toward him to say deflatingly, "A very standard catalog of S/M thematics, in fact;

I know that nothing
could be more ordinary
than such fantasies."

And I'm ashamed of *that*, too. There's not one single thing about them that I'm not ashamed of—as soon as I step outside their own, proprietary space. There, I love them.

I'm ashamed of their not being explainable to Shannon.

I'm afraid he won't be interested in them at all; leaving me out in the cold alone.

I'm also afraid he'll ask me—unlubricated—more

about them: there's not
a corner of the room far
enough to gaze at.

There's just a long pause.

"One thing I guess I do feel confident and practiced about, though: these fantasies stay in their place. They're just, exactly, fantasies. They don't connect with real life. The thought of acting them out with someone else, even in the most stylized scenes, feels completely beside the point of them.

"Of course, I used to fear that having such fantasies, and so compulsively, meant they'd inevitably leak into the rest of my life. Especially, that my relations with other people would be deformed by my being sadistic—or, much more likely, masochistic. Even though I *hate* violence, I *can't bear* shame or pain, mine or anyone else's. But looking at my life, at least over the past fifteen years or so, I've come to feel very sure that neither of those things is true."

Not in any way that he's picked up yet, Shannon agrees.

And anyhow, I say, it's kind of moot. I don't really have any more S/M fantasies. I don't really have any more autoerotic life at all.

Imperceptibly, inexorably, it all disappeared after I got cancer.

I realize I miss it.

This does pique Shannon's attention. "No fantasies? Where did they go, do you think?"

I shake my head hopelessly.

Then perk up. "But there was an interesting thing about fantasies that got dramatized for me. I hope this isn't too theoretical to say—it was an amazingly concrete effect. You know how the person in a fantasy feels like they're both you and not you at the same time? Well, it turned out that that was actually a requirement for the fantasy, at least for me.

"Because as my body got weirder with the treatment, I kept feeling that I had to choose, and couldn't. Either the girl in the fantasy would have one breast, or she would have two. Either she would have hair, or she would be bald. Apparently it couldn't be both ways. But if she was me, a bald woman with one breast, that ruined the fantasy—and if she wasn't me, wasn't marked in those ways, then that ruined the fantasy, too."

A funny thing, though: there are also ways that the cancer treatment did answer to my fantasies in a "warm" way, not in that horrifying, vengeful way.

Because it's important, for some reason, that the fantasies always have an institutional pretext—almost a bureaucratic one. They take place in a girls' school, a prison, or spy agency—always, always places with waiting rooms.

A lot of the punishment spaces are quasi-medical. Receptionists and undressing-rooms loom large. Doors open and doors close; people peer in. The "examination": fearful word!

The slant, withdrawn fellowship of waiting patients at the cancer clinic, the specific gravity of each thickened by dread: it's like the way people wait, about to be punished, in my fantasies. Names on the intercom, summonses to a fate, slash at the fragile pretense to privacy.

The unmarked new ones scanning, shyly, the ones experienced in indignity and loss.

> Other feelings stream
> back from the veterans, proud,
> ashamed, at once of

our practiced way with the awful routines.

"I'll tell you one moment when I felt it most—most intoxicatingly, almost, the touching of the two, utterly separate worlds.

"It was just, I think, before I started the six months of chemo; I was already worried about my bad veins. But some doctor needed some blood for something, so I went into the little anteroom where they take blood.

"It was occupied by a small late-middle-aged, prim, kind of severe Jamaican woman, that day. I've seen her there since.

"And as usual, it was hard to find a vein in my arm. She had to play darts for awhile, and eventually I told her—I knew this because I've always fainted easily—that I was about to faint.

"She seemed, well, irritated. The whole time, she'd made no eye contact with me.

"So she made me get up, and pushed me across the hallway to a long room, a long, dim, dormitory-like room, with beds on both sides, with movable screens separating the beds. I didn't know if anyone else was already in there.

"And she made me lie down, and she sat on the chair next to the bed. I could feel every pulse of her impatience.

"There was some rustling somewhere else in the room. Eventually my own heartbeats let go their grip of me, and I realized that someone was crying, trying hard not to be audible. Silent sobs, near silent muted hiccups. Somebody else somewhere was whispering. I could almost make out words.

"I could hear the moment when the nurse relaxed. When she realized that she'd never get blood out of me unless she could step away from the assembly line of her own temporality and simply stop. She silently put her hand over my hand on the bed.

"I realized something too: I had to stop hating her enough to give her the blood. Or it would all never end.

"I closed my eyes, withdrew my attention, tried to relax every muscle; tried to float freely away on the childish sensation of 'white bed,'

    to go ahead and
    faint, even, if to faint was
    how I'd surrender.

    I felt this was an
    initiation into
    my new, cancer life.

From her touch I could tell, now, that she meant to help me do it.

"And I wasn't sure it wasn't hallucinated (but it wasn't), when I heard a low voice somewhere—not near me—say rather distinctly to somebody else, 'Spread your legs.'"

———

"Can you *hear* all this at all? Are you getting any sense of how these things happen, for me?"

"Yes, I think I may
be. But unfortunately
we have to stop now."

————

I've already developed a strategy for "We have to stop now." In fact, most hours—not this one—I expect the sentence before it comes.

When it does come, I'll hop from the couch with an almost eager promptness. It's the same way, when I used to be in love with someone who wasn't in love with me, I would pantomime, "But I'll never be a burden to you." It signifies the supposed lightness of my demand and presence.

Shannon will sometimes take his time at such moments, though. His stockinged feet roll off our footrest, tuck into his loafers; his body balances up from the big, back-tilting chair to accompany me to the door.

To my great anxiety, there is even sometimes more to say.

This time he muses,
standing opposite me, his
demeanor friendly,

"It is interesting, though, that sexual fantasies can simply disappear. I wonder how people go about finding new ones to replace them."

I answer with a shrug, a sour moue: "Let me know if you find out."

"Well," he says, "I guess they'd have to explore the alternatives, no?

"Come to think of it, I wonder whether renting porn videos would be a good way. Just to try out a whole range of different kinds of fantasy, see what hit a nerve. You think?"

I expect I'm making a comical face of alarm as I turn to the door. Something like that.

He's going on: "They probably don't carry those at Blockbuster— but at Visart, maybe? Or magazines—that might feel more private,

less invasive. Especially if a particular fantasy didn't work. I'd probably try that, I suppose.

"Seems like a good thing to explore, anyway."

I don't know what my face is saying by this point, but my voice is
firm. I'll see you Thursday.

————————

By the time I get home, my unease has become palpable; by bedtime
it's grown to the kind of din that drowns things out. It's not till then I
see I'm more than uneasy: I'm frightened and enraged.

And it frightens me to *feel* rage, to have it reach into my senses so
deeply I can't see around it anymore, can't go on suspending it

> as I've suspended
> the worry about Shannon
> just being too dumb

these hours when I've splashed around so happily in his mild, hired
companionship. Too dumb or too nice—like, with no teeth, or at least
no tooth for me.

I need you *to change me* (I'm murmuring into the dark). Don't,
don't go being all stupid. You can't just let me drop.

But I'm certain he has done so.

————————

Those shrinks back in graduate school—how transparently they'd fish
for the transferential testimonials that were never forthcoming.

> "Maybe it was . . . your
> feelings about *me* . . . ?" Sorry,
> don't get your hopes up.

One of them did startle me into noting that my mother looked like her, but that was as far as it got.

Tonight, though, when I'm practically jumping out of my skin with "feelings about" my therapist, it's obvious that I can never utter them. What would I say? I could adore you, but you won't *think* enough? Don't you even *care* what garbage comes out of your mouth?

I might as well just say: be someone else.

Time to consult with experts—the scattered friends whose narratives of their own adventures in therapy convinced me to try it again in the first place. Exhausted the next day, I throw myself onto the phone, plunge into the e-waves.

In Amherst, Andy's no help. Laurie is a goddess to him; it could never seem possible for her to fail him. Ditto with Simon and his hieratic shrink in London. (It inspired me when Simon once said he loved Wednesdays because the *New Yorker* hit the stands and also he got to see this woman. My first clue that therapy and pleasure belong in the same breath.)

But Mary's been struggling for three years with her analyst in Boston, and she'll certainly recognize what I'm talking about. Mary says this to me: "I have never had the feeling of getting *anywhere* in this analysis—it's

almost true that I've
never felt anything but
sullen frustration.

But if I'd had a wish list when I started, it would have read, Stop smoking, Find a lover, Learn to exercise and enjoy having a body. And somehow—in no apparent relation at all to anything that happens between me and her—all those things have occurred."

Tim Gould is my e-mail addiction in Denver, and MR is the analyst he can see only once a week. I've known Tim for decades and recognize him as a top therapy maven.

"I thought Shannon listened well to the things I was saying," I write him, "—listening is actually a great skill of his, there's a wonderful quiet attentive look he has that is catnip to me—but, overcoming my anxiety about saying all this stuff, I think I made *him* anxious . . . at least, he said things at the end that were fatuous, overquick, conventional.

"I am disturbed by his seeming move into problem-solving mode as soon as sex enters the conversation, or something that could be classified—though *I* didn't classify it—as a 'sexual problem.' I'm off-balance about having initiated this discussion of sex at all, and don't see why he couldn't have guessed and respected that better. I keep wondering if maybe I wasn't supposed to talk about it, or not *now* for some reason, or . . .

"Night of long dreams (after 2 Benadryl, slept like a log, finally, but . . . a log that kept bursting into flame!). But I don't remember a one of them."

So it means something to me when Tim writes, "I think, from the little I can follow at the moment about your therapy, that you must be making progress.

Such a mild-mannered
fellow is Shannon, to be
stirring up the grounds

this much and this bitter already."

"I guess it made me
feel as if you hadn't been
hearing me at all,"

is what I'm saying when at last we see each other. "—You acting as if I could phone Sears, Roebuck and order myself new fantasies from the catalogue. Was that what it sounded like, my relation to sexual stuff? So free,

so arbitrary,
its root in me so shallow?
Can you have thought *that*? "

Shannon says he's not sure. "I guess there was something about the way you were talking about your S/M fantasies that sounded very abstract to me."

"*Abstract*? I don't see how you can be serious. It's such a huge, real fact to me. What I was saying about the cancer clinic, the institutional settings—that seemed abstract?"

"Yeah, to me it did."

He seems startled at my coming in sleepless, upset, speaking—after a few, tense commonplaces—in the tiny voice of my anger. My accusation: "I had the feeling you were even more anxious than I was at my wanting to talk about sex."

"Well," Shannon says equably, "that's very likely true. I expect it did make me anxious. So I probably wasn't listening very well."

This is disarming in the sense of stopping me in my tracks. Not in the sense of warming or reassuring, though his demeanor suggests it's supposed to be. It doesn't occur to me to ask, Why are you anxious about this? Instead, there's silence as I encounter the dusty roadblock of his answer and—swallow it.

THIS IS A COMPLICATED DYNAMIC. E TURNS TO SOMEONE FOR HELP OR GUID-ANCE OR UNDERSTANDING OF HERSELF OR A SITUATION SHE IS IN. THE PERSON DOESN'T OR CAN'T PROVIDE ADEQUATE, THOUGHTFUL HELP. I FEEL STUPID AND ALSO SAD THAT I CANNOT GIVE TO E WHAT SUPPORT I HAVE TO OFFER. E EXPERI-ENCES THE SITUATION AS A MORE BROAD-BASED ABANDONMENT, A FAMILIAR SITUATION IN WHICH SHE IS TOLD THAT SHE IS (TOO?) SMART OR ANOMALOUS, ON HER OWN, AND IS LEFT TO FIGURE IT OUT BY HERSELF. SHE EXPERIENCES THIS AS NOT JUST ABANDONMENT BUT ALSO AS INTENSE TIREDNESS. THE TOTAL DROPPEDNESS SHE FEELS SEEMS TO ME TO BE SOMETHING FROM HER PAR-ENTS—THAT OTHER PEOPLE MIGHT SAY THEY CAN'T HELP HER IN SOME SPE-CIFIC WAY BUT COULD STILL MAINTAIN CONTACT AND SUPPORT—BUT SHE DOESN'T EXPERIENCE THAT. ALSO, THE ONLY WAY OUT SEEMS TO BE HER INTEL-LECTUAL ACTIVITY—TO DO CONTINUAL SOLITARY WORK ON WHATEVER WITH HER MIND.

TELLS ME DREAM——AUSTRALIA——ADVENTURES GETTING TO ALICE SPRINGS——A
CONFERENCE——DISCUSSING *THE PICTURE OF DORIAN GRAY*, THEN AFTERWARD
"WE WILL BE READING THIS WONDERFUL ESSAY BY EVE SEDGWICK." SOMEONE
SAYS LET'S NOT DO THAT NOW, LET'S EVERYONE WRITE ON THE ROLE OF POSITIVE
AND NEGATIVE STEREOTYPES IN *DORIAN GRAY*. SHE IS IN A RAGE——A FIRE-
STORM IN HER HEAD ABOUT HOW IDIOTIC IT IS. THIS IS SO INTENSE THAT SHE
CANNOT WRITE ON THE QUESTION, AND MORE, BEGINS SAYING THE RAGE OUT
LOUD——FINALLY SAYS SHE IS ANGRY AND LEAVING AND NEVER COMING BACK
TO THIS CONFERENCE——THEY SAY THEY PAID HER WAY THERE AND SHE CAN'T
LEAVE——SHE DOES ANYWAY.

[NEXT SESSION] CHAGRIN ABOUT HAVING NARRATED DREAM, SAW AFTERWARD IT
WAS ABOUT ME AND THERAPY.

TALKS MORE @ LATE TEEN/EARLY MARRIAGE DEPRESSION WITH LOSS OF WRIT-
ING, SUPPRESSED ANGER, ANGUISH. NOT CLEAR WHY——SOME ASPECT SEXUALITY
VERY IMPORTANT HERE ESPECIALLY AS E NOT WANTING TO PARTICIPATE AS WELL
AS BEING UNCLEAR ABOUT IT IN GENERAL.

"When you said that S/M stuff sounded so abstract?" I ask Shannon
later, and he nods.

"Were you just referring to the fact that I wasn't offering details?
Because it's true I wasn't—but then you weren't exactly inviting them,
either. Or did you actually mean that you didn't get the flavor of it at
all? That it didn't get any purchase in your own feelings?"

After some thought he concludes, "The second thing."

"Really?"

"Uh-huh. I think so." A beat later, "You didn't think I meant abstract as in bad, did you? It was just abstract in the sense that—I didn't get it."

"No, I didn't think you were disapproving. But, well—well, if you didn't get that, then it seems to me that you must not vibrate to the chord of S/M practically at all. Because I think for anyone who did, what I was saying would have seemed very solid and resonant."

"I think you're probably right. That it would have, I mean. And also that I actually don't."

I feel as if he'd remarked casually that he doesn't breathe oxygen. Some people deeply believe that nobody can't be bought; my own deep conviction is that no one can be entirely unaroused around any scene of punishment.

Thinking it over that evening, I'm most surprised at one thing: I believe him. The sunniness of temper this implies to me—the unturbid current that must be his consciousness—challenges my notion of even what is human.

And yet our absolutely alien mental flows

debouch so freely
into the room where we meet!
A promise to me.

———

TALKS ABOUT FIRST SEXUAL OVERTURE BY HAL ABOUT 5–6 MO. INTO THEIR REL. HAD ADJUSTED TO HOPING IT WOULDN'T COME UP——DISAPPOINTED/SCARED. SHE IS CLEAR THAT SHE HAD NO INTEREST EITHER THEN (LACK OF RESPONSE/ FEELING INADEQUATE/GUILT/ANGER AFTER) OR EVEN AS MUCH YOUNGER CHILD. VAGUE FEELING, AS WITH MATERNAL GAZE, THAT SHE COULD NOT BE-LIEVE/ACCEPT THAT HIS INTEREST HAD ANYTHING TO DO WITH HER.

—But afterward there
is the big problem: how to
walk out of the room

and not still be in the space of old pain and hopelessness. I do see that it's an auspice of some kind of success, to be able to access that time so strongly when I've resisted turning my face toward it for so long—access it with Shannon, I mean. But I don't have—I doubt if I'm within a year of having—any resources for dealing with it outside his office, any at all.

I bring these thoughts up at the next session, so that at the end he's asking, "Do you think there's something more or different you need me to be doing so you'll feel more supported?"

And I'm angry at myself for not saying, Tell me what you've got on the menu. I mean, what I want to say is,

> Well if you wouldn't
> mind could you please just fold me
> up in your billfold,
>
> carry me like that
> around in your pocket for
> a couple of weeks?

I know the answer to that would not be a cheerful yes. So instead I immediately retreat to the realm of things I *can do myself* (like, things I can tell myself about him, or about me) that might make it all easier to take.

Whereas he might actually have had some concrete help to offer? And I'll never know because I don't ask, seemingly can't ask.

———————

WHEN SHE LEFT WED. SHE STILL FELT IN THE MIDST OF THE ANGUISH AND DE-PRESSION THAT SHE HAD TALKED @—UNCOMFORTABLY SO. TALKS TODAY ABOUT HOW THIS DEPRESSION PROGRESSED, FIRST WITH HER PRECIPITOUSLY FALLING IN LOVE WITH T.—UNREQUITED—THEN HAVING THE FIVE-YEAR AF-FAIR WITH K.C. MAYBE SIMPLY FINDING OUT SHE WASN'T TRAPPED IN THE MAR-

RIAGE SITUATION WAS ENOUGH TO ALLEVIATE THE DEPRESSION——AND ALSO
FINDING OUT THAT SHE DID NOT LOSE HAL IN THE PROCESS.

——————

FEELING MUCH BETTER TODAY. TELLS ME ABOUT THE PANDA RITUALS SHE AND
HAL HAVE. THESE DEVELOPED AROUND THE TIME WE HAVE BEEN DISCUSSING
AND, AMONG OTHER THINGS, ALLOWED HER TO FEEL MAGNETIC, RARE, AND
VALUED EVEN WHILE GAUCHE AND UNSEXUAL ETC. IN INTERACTIONS WITH
HIM. BOTH OF THEM SEE ASPECTS OF THEMSELVES IN THIS ANIMAL. STILL IN
THE LATE TEEN—EARLY 20S PERIOD: THIS TIME ABOUT HOW SHE WENT INTO
MARRIAGE IN THE SAME "DIVING IN" FASHION WITH ITS HYPER AND DESPER-
ATE EDGE THAT CHARACTERIZED HER IN CHILDHOOD.

——————

DREAM OF LIVING SOMEWHERE WHERE SHE HAS A COLLIE WHICH SHE IS TO
CARE FOR BUT WHICH IS INJURED. SHE KEEPS FORGETTING THAT SHE IS SUP-
POSED TO DO SOMETHING FOR IT AND THEN REMEMBERING. ——THERE WAS A
COLLIE AT THE COMMUNE WHERE SHE AND HAL FIRST LIVED WHICH WAS A
BLUE COLLIE SO SHE CALLED IT "MELANCHOLY." SHE SAYS THAT SHE OFTEN HAS
DREAMS OF NOT REMEMBERING TO CARE FOR SOMETHING OR SOMEONE,
WHICH USUALLY INVOLVE THE DEATH OR THREATENED DEATH OF WHATEVER IT
IS. RELATES THE DREAM TO MICHAEL'S HAVING HAD ANOTHER PAINFUL ATTACK
OF CORNEAL ABRASION. SHE TALKS ABOUT THE CARETAKING SHE MUST HAVE
GOTTEN AS A CHILD WHERE SHE REMEMBERS HESITANTLY GOING TO GET IN
BED WITH HER PARENTS IF SHE WAS QUITE SCARED IN THE NIGHT. THIS TIES
SOME TO HER SISTER ALWAYS GETTING INTO BED WITH HER.

4

We get into a talk about timidity, my timidity, and how the ways that he usually knows how to "encourage" somebody don't work with me. Instead they cause bristling or sensations of being dropped. I tell him one example, from a couple of meetings ago— ". . . So, thinking about it, of course my first impulse was, 'How can I make him stop acting this way?' But then I realized it also raised some *interesting questions* . . ."

"Oh, no, don't give up on how to make me stop acting this way!"

There's something about these What-are-we-going-to-do-about-Eve conversations that delights me. It's as if Shannon and I are Eve's parents, half exasperated and half impressed with her resistance to the pedagogies we're used to administering. I guess our daughter is really exceptional, huh?

Or maybe less like being her parents than like (one of the most fantasy-ridden, occult scenes of childhood) the parent-teacher conference.

Say I'm the parent,
in the sense of being the
expert on the child

—while Shannon, the teacher, can see her in a different context. He's the one with the methodologies, "skills," comparative frameworks to be bent, adapted, exceeded, or even broken.

"What kind of a narrative," I want to know, "are we trying to construct—or do we think we need to construct—about Eve's history? I mean, what's the purpose of it, what do we want from it?"

As opposed (I don't say) to the transferential thing, which seems to grow like a weed from one day to the next.

"Well," he says, "when I think about how I want you to *turn out* different, the thing about blaming yourself all the time is near the top of the list."

I'm not surprised at that—it's pretty obvious—but am a bit surprised he'll admit to keeping a list of how he wants me different.

But he also says

he wants me to have
a more continuous sense
of moving through time.

"Less spastic" is his gracious description. "To see yourself being more of the same person."

Not identical,
not grappled tight to myself,
just floating onward.

"I know I promised
not to 'mirror' you, but I
can't help" (Shannon says

one day) "remarking
how I hear so much sadness
in the things you say."

It's without sadness,
but with interest, that he
does so. "—How many

questions I want to
ask you about that sadness!"
     I probably smirk

while saying something
deprecating about my
awful self-pity,

but seriously
he says self-pity's not the
note he's tuned in to.

"Well," I tell him, "ask."
"Well, then," he says to me, "first,
     what's it all about?

What is it you haven't thought to tell me? I mean, is someone actually
dying, back there in Dayton, Ohio? Is there some obvious way you're
learning these things about death and loss? What is it meaning to
you—loss, death? Or what does it mean in your family? You don't have
to answer all these questions at once, but that's what's on my mind."

———

But nobody's dying. Absolutely no one, I'm sure of it. My grandparents all live till after I've left home. My mother—well, she has a mis-
carriage or a stillbirth in between me and my little brother, and I used
to wonder whether she might have been depressed about that, and if
I kind of introjected it. But David asked my father about it once, and
he said, if anything they were relieved by the loss of the baby.

Shannon looks discontented. "I'm sure there's more to figure out about that one. But somehow I want something else to have happened, something big and awful and early. Course maybe I'm wrong, but I want to hold out for something on that scale."

"I'm dubious. If there was, I have to say I just don't know about it." Of course I've wondered this for a long time. "I'd like to know about it, I think I would. But what it feels like is that I just *am* this way; I think I've always been. Certainly as long as I remember. Sadness is such a groundtone for me. I almost only feel like myself when I'm sad."

This answer, plain common sense to me, doesn't make Shannon happy. "It isn't that I'm doubting you *are* this way, no. Or even that you have been for a long time. But here's a principle I really do tend to believe—that for every effect there's a cause. You could even say a proportionate cause, if you don't mind sounding a little mechanical. So when someone says, 'I just am that way,' I get extra interested."

Now something about
the thought of this is very
exciting to me

but that doesn't mean
I'm sitting still for it, I
know better than *that*:

"What counts as 'proportionate,' though?" I'm asking with teacherly patience. "Doesn't it depend on the person, on how they're already put together? So that the 'cause' of a big effect could be something that, from the outside, looks big or looks tiny . . ."

Like, I'm thinking, the spankings we used to get.

"Oh, sure. That's why I want to get to know someone well—see more about the scale their emotional life is on to begin with."

I'm stubborn (another way I've "always been"). "But another thing is that it seems—for all the sadness and morbidity inside me as a child—as though really it wasn't till I was an adult that I genuinely experienced loss. Never mind death. It's seemed so *new* when it's come to me as an adult."

"Tell me a few times that it has?" Willingly, quietly, disconcertingly to me in this case, Shannon slips gears. "Has it, has it come as death or as other things?"

I'm quiet too for several seconds, thinking, organizing. "It's come in several forms. I'll tell you the ones I think were the worst for me, the ones from which I think that I know now what loss does feel like. They're very disproportionate—at least with each other. I don't think most of them have the shape you're thinking of as *big* and *awful*. Though they've been that way for me."

"Don't mind me. Don't let me make you not say anything you're going to say."

———

There was some death. I was eighteen when my Grandpa died suddenly—but at least he was "old," though I realize now not very old. Then, two years later, Hal's best friend was blown up by a land mine in Vietnam.

Then a year after that, Frank Rosenblatt, Hal's professor who owned the farmhouse where we were living, died in a boating accident. It was a commune where he was the kind of absent-minded-scientist daddy. That was the very most shocking, the most completely out of the blue, and he was someone we loved who was also a central person in our everyday lives. There's a way that after that I never stopped knowing how abruptly absolutely anything could be lost.

"Three very sudden deaths, so sudden I almost didn't process them at all. —That's what I thought death was like, sudden numbing shocks, full of horror but almost exciting—I mean what I thought someone else's death was like, until AIDS."

Quiet again, thinking what to say about the kinds of loss the epidemic has brought. But Shannon is also quiet, slipping back another gear— "And the losses that weren't people dying? Those are the ones that feel disproportionate?"

I try to clear my head for it.

"Yes. So much it's actually hard to say them."

Shannon offers, in a playful tone and it seems to me absurdly, "I

once had a patient who had a particular thing he couldn't tell me until I promised to cover my eyes and not peek till he was finished." He
smiles in apparent self-appreciation.

> Flare of my rage and
> mortification at this
> buffoonish offer—
>
> infantile as the
> offer's infantilizing.
> My put-out silence,
>
> till, defocusing,
> I'm back in chemo, the shock
> of losing my hair
>
> ("the breast was *nothing!*"—
> a good thing, too, of course, since
> the hair does grow back

but not till after six months of a monstrosity from which there was no

> hiding myself); or
> I'm back in graduate school
> failing my orals
>
> —Injury, insult;
> in my Dickensian school-
> room of a brain, don't
>
> they add up alike
> to violent hemorrhage
> of the stuff of self,

or like the guillotine of awfulness that was the sheer end, four years
ago, of a friendship as intimate and passionate to me as Michael's—

"That abruptly. No warning. Every bit of me that was lodged in him was lost to me, I guess forever. And it was very graphic: every bit of Benj that was lodged in me stayed in me. It had nowhere else to go. But now it hated me, it seemed to hate me with every molecule of its being, of his."

"You're talking about stuff in your own head."

"In mine, yeah. That was when I felt in an almost hallucinatory way, for months and months, what it really meant, my inability to identify with myself.

"—And I guess I'd never been quite hated before."

"You've spoken to him since?"

"Never could." The couple of times I've seen him, all I could feel was, If looks could kill . . .

Then when I got the
diagnosis it was like,
"Oh. Of course. They can."

———

Or like the loss of poetry, I tell him.

"You're a poet? Or you were?"

Oh, yes. I'm stunned—for how can he not know? It was my first vocation, first identity—from early childhood on into my thirties. (When my grandmother lost her memory and didn't know our names or relationships, she still mouthed, pointing at me, "The poet?") Poetry both my first love, I guess, and first self—always with the most excruciating blockages—gone now for years. Really gone for a decade. I can't think about it; I don't; when I used to, it would make me crazy. I don't know if it was depression that drove this muse away or if it was the long rocky strand of her loss that made depression.

"I do know I'm incredibly fortunate in my second love. Never expected to be able to pour my self and energies into critical writing, have them so answered . . ."

———

DREAM—WITH A GROUP OF PEOPLE BUT E IS PLAYING APART FROM THEM.
THERE IS A GAME INVOLVING SOME DEXTERITY AND SOME THINKING SKILL.
SHE IS CONTENTEDLY PLAYING EVEN THOUGH SHE IS LOSING. THEN SOMEONE
SAYS TO HER THAT THERE IS A RULE THAT AFTER YOU LOSE SO MANY TIMES (6?)
YOU CAN NEVER PLAY THE GAME AGAIN. SHE IS CRUSHED. THROUGH THE REST
OF THE DREAM SHE TRIES TO FIGURE OUT IN HER OWN MIND IF IT IS REALLY A
RULE, WHERE THE RULE COMES FROM, IF THESE PEOPLE ACTUALLY TAKE IT SERI-
OUSLY. MOST DIFFICULT IS THAT SHE FEELS SHE CANNOT ARTICULATE HER
QUESTIONS TO THE OTHER PEOPLE—IF THEY DO TAKE THE RULE SERIOUSLY
SHE WON'T EVER BE ABLE TO PLAY IT AGAIN, IF THEY DON'T SHE WILL LOOK LIKE
AN IDIOT FOR ASKING. ALSO SHE IS ASHAMED OF BEING SO UPSET ABOUT A
GAME. SHE HAS TO DEAL WITH ALL OF IT INSIDE HERSELF. /// FEW ASSOCIATIONS
BUT THE SENSE OF SOME IMPORTANCE TO THE DREAM. I ASK HOW HER PARENTS
WOULD RESPOND WHEN SHE WAS UPSET. SHE SAYS FATHER MIGHT EXPLAIN USE-
FULLY OR OVEREXPLAIN, MIGHT IGNORE. HER MOTHER WOULD SAY SOMETHING
OBLIQUE, PARADOXICAL, OR UNCONCERNEDLY REASSURING WHICH WAS NOT
COMFORTING. MY QUESTION IS THAT THIS SEEMS LIKE A COMMON CHILDHOOD
EXPERIENCE OF FINDING OUT THAT THERE WAS A RULE YOU DIDN'T KNOW.
THEN WHY IS THIS SO TRAUMATIC FOR HER—HOW DO YOU MAKE THIS EXPE-
RIENCE TRAUMATIC FOR A KID?

A beastly few weeks of Durham weather, and my image for the therapy is a kind of tepid bath (I love tepid baths). "Tepid" referring both
to the often insipidity of our actual exchanges, and to the new sense of
a possibility of refreshment.

> —Bath into which I
> slowly lower my great bulk,
> to be supported

in some medium less human than "holding" (in Winnicott's famous
image of therapeutic relation) would suggest.

That is, there's something about being *impersonally* held; and not impersonal because Shannon is so cool (he's so uncool!)—but exactly because, I guess, of how the substance of most of the things he says seems to lap, quite consistently, just below my threshold of "interest."

WE DISCUSS OFF-BALANCE MOMENTS OF CHILDHOOD. SHE RECALLS A SITUATION OF BEING EXPECTED TO TAKE A WALK WITH THE REST OF THE FAMILY—AT FIRST THINKING THAT SHE HAD A CHOICE BUT SOON FINDING OUT THAT THE WALK WAS MANDATORY. SHE MENTIONS PART OF THIS "WALK" ISSUE BEING HER POSITION IN THE FAMILY AS THE FAT KID.

"Fat kid! No. I might, thinking back about some of those pictures, go so far as . . . 'chubby.' (Remember chubby?) But, no; I'd really have to say that for your family to think of the kid in those pictures as fat—that verges on delusional."

"Yeah, but what you're seeing is the distance from how fat I am now. That wasn't what they were looking at then."

When I say this he almost lunges at me. "*No*, that is *not* what I'm seeing. To view that kid as fat is really—really to be at the very edge of being in contact with reality." Then he asks if there was a system of scapegoating, or any such family mechanism, to which I could attribute this group delusion.

I have an account of this: beginning with my father's father as the designated sufferer from "weight problems," a role devolving onto my father, further devolving (when I come on the scene) onto me.

"And you could understand when you were a kid how this mechanism was working?"

"Oh, yes. I understood it very clearly as far back as I can remember."

"And was there a part of you, do you think, that refused to believe it all?"

"Yeah, I think there must have been—from the fact of my having survived even as little damaged as I have been."

He nods, pleased. "There was a part of you that could say—'Wait a minute, I'm not fat at all! I'm just fine!'"

Me. Rather bitterly. "Well, I think—actually, I hope—there was a part of me that was saying, Yes, I *am* fat, and I'm great."

"You don't think it ever occurred to you that you weren't?"

"No. Again, I infer this—even from my having gotten so fat later, I infer that, yes, I did identify with that sense of myself. And that the issue was never fat or not fat, but— given fat—worth something or worth nothing?

"Always, I think, always, my body was going to appear as a problem. I remember how miserably I used to think about it, between, say, eight and fourteen—the years when I had braces, *and* my folks got me contact lenses when I didn't especially want them, *and* there was all the talk about when would be the right time for me to have a nose job. Never mind the fat stuff. It was so clear to me that every single thing about my body was unacceptable."

Also clear that the me my folks were seeing was different from the me I was experiencing.

Not really because I seemed acceptable to myself (sometimes I did, but often not); but because I thought they saw me as infinitely malleable—as some perfectible thing—putty. But I knew I was a person already;

quite simply I was
not malleable in that
way. There I just was.

"And you were able to feel pretty secure in that."

"Oh, no. No. No. No, there were layers—layers on layers—and in a lot of them I thought I could become anything; could yield to anything; *was* malleable, unformed, was scarcely there at all."

Then, after a while, I murmur something inaudible.

"What?" he asks sharply.

"It enrages me," I say louder.

"Well, *good*! I was sitting here wondering if there was anything I could possibly feel about this besides angry—anything that would let me be even remotely in synch with you . . ."

––––––––

A moment's realization, startlingly clear. "I've figured out what it means when I complain to you about things," I tell him. "Or to anybody. When I tell you how bad it is, how hard I've worked at something, how much I've been through, there is only one phrase I want to hear.
   "Which is:

'That's enough. You can
   stop now.'
             Stop: living, that is.
   And *enough*: hurting.

"Like, 'I didn't realize how hard it was for you; you've done well; you've been through plenty; you're excused."

––––––––

That's enough; you can stop now. Isn't this the blessing into whose enfolding arms every complaint of suffering bounds—in its dreams?
   At least, it means that in my native land.
   Five miles across the border, phrasebooks say, it's different.
   There, it's a way that parents calm their kids.

––––––––

I'm trying to think of other things that "that's enough, you can stop now" could have meant—aside from, yes, you don't have to live anymore. I come to a scenario: a kid getting a bit hyper, showing off, talking loud, acting funny or something, who is—no, *not* told to cut it out—but, instead, rebuked (deliberately or absent-mindedly) by being, after a certain point, ignored.

So the kid is somehow stuck in this behavior without having anyone to let them know: that's enough, you can stop now.

———

WE END UP TALKING ABOUT HOW IMPORTANT IN HER FAMILY IT WAS NOT TO SAY THINGS IN THE WRONG TONE OF VOICE. THIS STARTS WITH E TALKING ABOUT HOW HARD IT ALWAYS IS FOR HER TO ASK FOR ANYTHING SHE NEEDS, HOW CAREFUL AND LONG-PLANNED ANY REQUEST ALWAYS IS. IT IS IMPORTANT NOT TO WHINE, NOT TO INDICATE THAT YOU HAVE BEEN SUFFERING FOR LACK OF SOMETHING, NOT TO SOUND AS IF YOU EXPECT TO GET WHAT YOU ASK FOR, NOT TO PRESUME, NOT TO . . . I FRAME THIS IN TERMS OF FINE-TUNING THE CHILDREN'S CHORUS.

———

There's a beguiling gravity in Shannon's listening mien. He is a vastly different listener from what he is as a talker (and he's not at all the silent type). He listens with sobriety and, I would say, delicacy; while, speaking, he'll disconcertingly act like a sacred clown

> or just a buffoon—
> the sonorous, nasal voice,
> broad facial gesture.

Now the gap between these two Shannons is the kind of gap I'm most prone to tumble into. "It's like," I say to him when I tell him about this, "if you have sex with somebody and they're totally different, during sex, from the way you're used to seeing them. As though you're allowed to see a different person. And then you have to figure out if you can elicit that new person at other times, at least the tokens and memories of them; and you get drawn in . . ."

For some reason this speaks powerfully to him. "*I* do that," he says, "and *you* do that. But do you think everybody does that? What do you think it's about?" I do assume that everybody does it. But maybe I'm wrong?

Something else about that listening mien. I feel a longing for the absorbency of it. For the fact that it carefully, deliberately won't (I expect, won't ever) visibly register . . . anything but attention. Won't register excitement, hurt, anxiety, threatenedness, arousal.

> All of these things move
> tracelessly inward, to be
> remembered—or not;

to be produced again at the "right" time or just another time (and produced as if they'd always been obvious, somehow).
The only flag of emotion that this

> listening face of
> Shannon ever displays: a
> thick, violet blush.

FROM A WHILE AGO E HAS LATCHED ONTO THE CONCEPT THAT SHE IS SOMEONE WHO FEELS NEED TO MAKE OTHERS SMARTER—THIS COMING FROM RECOGNITION THAT SHE FELT RESPONSIBLE FOR ELICITING MY INTELLIGENT INTEREST. SHE HAS ASKED SEVERAL PEOPLE ABOUT THIS AND GOT CONFIRMATION EXCEPT FROM ONE COLLEAGUE WHOM SHE CLEARLY FEELS SHE HAS MADE SMARTER. IS REALLY SHAKEN BY THIS BUT STILL HOLDS ON TO THE CONCEPT OF HERSELF AS MAKING PEOPLE SMARTER. (E: "MAKE THEM SMART" = SPANK THEM?) RELATES BACK TO THE EARLY ENGAGEMENT PROBLEMS WITH HER MOTHER. BUT FROM THE DEFLATION BROUGHT ABOUT BY HER FRIEND'S DISCONFIRMATION, SHE FOCUSES ON THE GRANDIOSITY IN THE CONCEPT. MY COMMENT IS THAT NORMAL DEVELOPMENT SEEMS TO ME TO MOVE FROM GRANDIOSITY TO DISILLUSIONMENT, BUT IN HER CASE IT MAYBE MOVES TO HER TRYING TO CONSOLIDATE AND MAKE PRACTICAL HER, SOMEWHAT GRANDIOSE, WAY OF SEEING HERSELF.

I try and try but never succeed in getting Shannon interested in genius—or even in "brilliance." It's an area of possibility and pathos that leaves him cold. The furthest he'll go, in his blandness, is describing someone as "really bright."

Talent, however, fascinates him. And even better, *talents*—the difference and specificity of talents, even in the same person. He loves to trace the shape and unexpected uses of a talent.

> When I try on this
> habit of his, I love it.
> Farewell to genius!
>
> Hello, welcome, to
> my talent and my talents,
> some big—some little.

I've always loved the parable about the talents, anyway; always craved narratives where the young talent receives nurture in figuring out what talent it *is*. But in Shannon's inquisitive notion of many particular talents, it seems that a person's talents also involve the many characteristic ways in which they might be stupid or resistant. Giving a person some license to ponder

> even blockages,
> yes, even block-headedness—
> and overreaching
>
> and pretentiousness—
> and solicit their dumbness
> with love and patience.

When Shannon pushes the story toward adolescence, I love evoking Girl Scout camp, age twelve—getting a crush on one of the counselors; cutting my thumb with a knife while whittling soap and being deliciously fussed over and comforted; being inept at all the camp-type activities but still feeling as if I was making a place for myself with sheer, dorky Evie-ness; unexpectedly and unpreparedly getting my period in the middle of all this, very embarrassed but, again, fussed over, enjoying that; intimacy (trading stories about grownup things: death, sex) with a baby butch in my tent; early experiments with the pleasure of voices—mine silvery—in the dark.

I can contrast this lusciously homosocial space with the strained, puppet-like heterosexual impositions and self-impositions of junior high school.

Shannon remarks, "But it doesn't really sound as if there was anything sexual about this Girl Scout camp space."

"It doesn't?"

"I mean, it wasn't coed or anything, not like your school."

Unmistakable manifestations of impatience from the sofa.

"What you're describing about the camp, it sounds like that has to do with nurturance, really, not with sexuality . . ."

"Like these have nothing to do with each other?"

"Well, sure. But you need to make it clearer, then, what kind of sexual charge some of this might have had, what it felt like to you."

"It felt like—a good image for it is—I mean, *you wouldn't know about this*, but imagine what it feels like when you're about to get your period. There's an almost familiar tug, a hand closing, in your abdomen . . . You don't particularly associate it with your cycle, at least if you're really young . . . It feels more like your own self-presence, but more so. Later, of course, it turns into ordinary pain,

> but before being
> cramps, it's this pull, as if of
> excess gravity—

that you *could* read as sexual; but you could also *not*. That's the best image I have for being at camp.

"Whereas what was going on at school—it was (at least for me it was) more like trying to learn a language. And except for English, I'm awful at languages."

———

I find only half a dozen teenage snapshots to show—and mostly they don't show much. Shannon's words for this body and face are matronly, masklike, and I guess I can see why. But one he connects with, showing me under a tree with my father's dad, whom I look just like, and inimitably out-of-it.

It occurs to me to say: something I see in that picture we haven't talked about and might sometime—that's the notion of "sweet." I think "sweet" is probably pretty important.

Shannon taking off his thick glasses, staring closely at the snapshot. Then, to my surprise, springing nimbly from his chair.

"I'm kind of knock-kneed, so I'm not sure I can do this, but . . ." he says, and I see he's studying the picture and trying to pretzel into just the same posture—feet in a sort of third position, chin and eyes down to the right, hands clasped in a twist behind the back.

Having done so: "Sweet!" he announces. "Sweet! You're right! It feels sweet! I had no idea, just looking at it, quite how sweet it was! But I can feel it in the tension across my shoulders, all the way down into my back; kind of smiling,

> looking off to the
> side. Yes, *sweet* is what I feel!"
> Shannon bewitching.

———

RETURNS TO ABOVE IN THAT SHE TALKS A LOT ABOUT 7TH GRADE AND THE DIS-
MISSAL OF HER FRENCH TEACHER AFTER BEING ARRESTED FOR SOLICITING IN A
MEN'S ROOM. THIS INVOLVES A LOT OF THEMATIC MATERIAL. SHE HAD NOT
KNOWN THAT, AS HER MOTHER EXPLAINED IT, THERE WERE MEN WHO LOVED

OTHER MEN THE WAY MOST MEN LOVE WOMEN. THIS CAUGHT HER IMAGINA-
TION AND SHE BEGAN READING INSATIABLY IN THE AREA, BUT ONLY ABOUT GAY
MEN——IT WAS ONLY LATER THAT SHE LEARNED ABOUT LESBIANS. THIS INTEN-
SITY WAS SOME PROPELLED BY HER CHAGRIN AT HAVING MISREAD THE FRENCH
TEACHER SO COMPLETELY——HER PERCEPTUAL ACUMEN HAVING FAILED HER.
YET IN THE LOOKING INTO AND LEARNING ABOUT IT HER FASCINATION WITH
IMPLICIT THEMES WAS ENGAGED AND SHARPENED. IT ALSO PROVIDED SOME-
THING OF AN OUT IN HER STRUGGLE WITH THE HETEROSEXUAL DEMANDS OF
ADOLESCENCE——THAT THERE COULD BE SOMETHING OTHER THAN THE TRADI-
TIONAL HETERO RELATIONS, AND MEN WHO MIGHT HAVE AN INTEREST IN
WOMEN OTHER THAN THE TRADITIONAL ONE. WHAT STRIKES ME MOST HERE IS
EARLY ABILITY TO TURN A SITUATION OF PROHIBITION AND RIGID EITHER/OR
INTO A NEW INTEREST THAT IS ELASTIC, PRODUCTIVE, EXCITING FOR E'S VIEW
OF WORLD. BUT HOW TO RELATE TO HER JR HS DEPRESSION??

Folk explanations for the onset of bad depression at thirteen: "First, raging hormones, of course," I say. "Imagine having all that PMS, not even knowing what it *was*.

"But also, junior high was so different; it seemed to offer so much wider a canvas for action, attention getting, achievement. Of course I couldn't not want it. But of course I couldn't get much of it, either—I wasn't pretty, or interpersonally skillful, or athletic or self-confident— and I think each time I tried and failed, I would batter myself for having been tempted off-center, for losing hold of my tenuous sense of myself. As though the floorboards of my self-esteem would periodically just collapse. And now I'm wondering if this was the first time that happened to me, at least on a regular basis.

"As if maybe, up till then, the practice of constant masturbation had actually succeeded in keeping my anxiety under control. But suddenly I was just flooded."

I add, "It's awfully striking how much the thread of a self, for me, seems to have been tied up with all this masturbating."

"Striking to me, too," Shannon says. "It seems to have been what made you feel safe—almost what made you feel held."

"You mean that's odd, because I'm alone then?" Shannon nods. "But it's true being alone does exactly that for me.

A summer morning,

waking up in my own good

time, with my cool skin,

a writing project waiting when I get around to it: for me, these are the real elements of heldness on a day-to-day basis. More even than being held by another person.

"Yes," I add after a while, "I do see that it's funny there isn't another person on the scene."

And after another while, "What if we say this about the junior high depression: up to then, however off-center I might have felt when I was around other people, at least being by myself meant being safe *with* myself. But suddenly, being so savage to myself and so turbulent, I lost that sense of sanctuary. Being by myself became as dangerous as being with other people. Probably even more so."

RETURN TO PHOTOS ESP. OF 13 Y/O GIRL SMILING, ARMS OUTSTRETCHED.

I am lovely in this photo, taken by my father. On the edge of a chair, but sort of flying toward the camera, my arms spread wide, looking nubile, mouth ecstatically open, eyes almost closed—quite radiant.

It looks like an awfully depressed person, momentarily exalted, who is about to crash in some disastrous way. Today we get arrested at this picture. And the more he wants me to talk about why I find it so scary, the more mistrustful I feel about why *he* finds it strange for me to find it so.

—and why, I presume, he also finds it so attractive. In fact, I finally accuse him of finding it attractive *because* the young woman in it looks so off-balance and exploitable— "Like Marilyn Monroe, when what people can't resist is the incandescence of her being so unstable."

ASTOUNDING TO HER TO HAVE FOUND HERSELF SO MISTRUSTING AND RESENT-
FUL OF ME AS SOON AS WE BEGAN TALKING ABOUT HER AT AGE 13 IN ABOVE
PICTURE. STILL FEELING THIS WAY TODAY—SURPRISED I CANNOT SEE THE UN-
HAPPINESS, FRAGILITY IN THE GIRL IN THE PIC. IN RELATION TO PIC SHE VAC-
ILLATES BETWEEN NOT RECOGNIZING THE GIRL AS HERSELF AND KNOWING HER
WITH THE KNOWLEDGE OF WHAT SHE WILL GO THROUGH IN NEXT SEVERAL
YEARS AS WELL AS HOW SHE IS COMING INTO THIS TIME. IS ABLE TO CONVEY TO
ME HOW CHAOTIC AND DANGEROUS SHE FEELS THESE YEARS ARE FOR HER.
ONLY PARTLY BECAUSE OF THE TURBULENCE OF ADOLESCENCE, MORE BECAUSE
SHE COMES INTO THESE YEARS WITHOUT A SECURE GRASP ON WHO HER SELF IS.

It's hard to credit how, with *one single* step over the line from kid pictures into puberty, I'm turned into a person who doesn't trust Shannon, and near enough even doesn't *like* him. Me stunned and frightened.

But also, "I'm remembering my interest around then in craziness and crazy people. It seemed so plausible to me that I might not wind up a sane adult myself.

"And there was such a wide range of states (being angry, sad, tipsy, exuberant, self-conscious—almost anything but perfectly tranquil) that seemed, when I experienced them, like gaping doors to insanity.

"The whole preoccupation seems so alien now!"

Now, when I've traveled far enough to recognize depression, not psychosis, as my companion for the journey.

—But looking at that picture with Shannon, with the instant turbulence it brings to our relation, seems a direct pipeline back to that time;

also I notice
the angle of the photo
emphasizes this

girl's breasts quite a lot
and I'm picturing Shannon
appreciating

the new, soft, alien
curves from my father's point of
view behind the lens

(he admits to this
identification!) while
for me, even when

I had the two breasts
I kept forgetting them. They
weren't there for me.

THIS DISCUSSION DOES NOT RESOLVE OUR RELATIONS NOW OR MAYBE MY RELA-
TION TO THIS GIRL AS YET.

———————

TALKING ABOUT HOW SEVERAL ELEMENTS OF SEXUALITY GOT EXPRESSED IN THE
FAMILY. E'S MOTHER SEEMS TO HAVE PRESENTED A DESIRED AND OFT-SPOKEN-
ABOUT PICTURE OF PREPUBESCENT GIRLHOOD FOR HER FATHER IN HER SLIGHT
STATURE AND GIRLISH FIGURE. THIS "ARRESTING" OF THEIR SEXUAL RELATION-
SHIP IN THE PRE-ADOLESCENT YEARS WAS MIXED WITH E'S MOTHER'S IGNOR-
ING OF E'S MASTURBATORY ACTIVITY AND WITH THE MOTHER'S INSERTION OF A
LITERARY SEXUALITY INTO THE FAMILY'S EVERYDAY LIFE, BUT SOMEHOW UNRE-
LATED TO THE FAMILY MEMBERS. THIS SEEMS TO ME TO BE A HYSTERICAL PIC-
TURE—FILLED WITH DISSOCIATED ELEMENTS, WHICH INCLINES E TO THE
FRAGMENTATION WHICH SHE HAS IN HER OWN SEXUALITY. I AM INTERESTED
IN THE EFFECTS GROWING CHILDREN HAVE ON THIS STABLE, PRE-ADOLESCENT
PARENTAL PICTURE.

"What do we call it, your mom's quality?" Shannon asks. "Girlishness? Boyishness?"

"Kiddishness," I suggest.

I'm struck by the promise and interest—he, by the fragility of such a gender placement: fragile for the project of raising kids through puberty and beyond.

It is simply true—I mean it's true in how I still perceive all three of us kids, as well as in the family image repertoire—that puberty was seen as catastrophic for the mental balance, the sociability, and the physical appeal of each of us.

Shannon's been brooding over the web of knowing, allusive, sexualized language my mother throws over her accounts of things. All the worldly relish and double-entendre go oddly with her Peter Pan innocence. My own obsessive site of brooding is what must have been her predicament in those years in the fifties: the cozy and joined-at-the-hip, but only fragmentarily sexual, Marriage and Family setup; the likely pressure of near-unconscious panic and claustrophobia about all this; and the need for a sense that *somewhere, out there in the world* (if not here in the family) were all kinds of practices, not to be named exactly, but to afford an epistemologically unstable shimmer of allusion and, sort of, possibility.

"I think my mother and I approach sexual things similarly: this sturdy, basically incredulous, latency-marked sense of clinical curiosity, funniness, and distance—along with fascination. As though basically neither of us can quite believe we aren't making the whole thing up out of our heads!" A certain

gaily denuding
brutalism about sex: my
mother's *kiddishkeit*.

Shannon's interested in the sexual advice my brother says he got from Daddy. "You'll have lots of strange and even upsetting feelings and thoughts," David was told, "but just remember, they're only feelings and thoughts, so don't feel guilty about them or feel you have to completely suppress them."

Then there's the kind of advice my mother gave me. Yes, on the one hand, a diffuse sense of odd sexualities *out there* that might be okay—but that don't have anything to do with things I might myself feel.

On the other hand, that I'd need to be unrestingly cautious about not being the victim of other people's—men's—sexual desires. Not because I might share or be responsive to them, either. At least as I heard it, her presumption was that my own romances would be in my head, but could be misunderstood or fake-misunderstood by men as physical.

How well I learned it,

her lexicon of
hypervigilance—men whose
wives *don't understand*

them, or who want to
show you etchings, or just "want
to lie down and take

a nap beside you"
on the couch, or get you drunk
or into the back

seat. However, "If
you let men touch you, they won't
keep respecting you."

Maybe my pickup
of this advice was skewed by
my *rage for respect*?

Of course these were the years before *Roe v. Wade*: the real-world sanctions against sexual expression, for a young woman, *were* crushing.

Still, Shannon remarks: how social it was, the advice I got, when David's was so inward-looking. He was to be the subject of a sexuality; I, a reluctant object or a knowing, psychologizing, yet comically unimplicated chronicler of it.

My skittish mother!
The wisdom she passed on to
an anxious daughter:

"Always dress for a
job interview as if you
didn't need a job.

Learn how to type, but
never let anybody
know that you know how."

We're back in the pink room of childhood masturbation, and Shannon is gesturing at something that's come up before: what he seems to think of as my parents' "neglect" in letting me spend so much time in my room jerking off over that period of years.

I'm not sure I understand it right, what he really thinks of this. But his line of thought alarms me, and this time I'm skinless enough to jump in.

"You know I'm very protective of that child's privacy to masturbate. I don't think of it as neglect at all." My eyes brimming.

Shannon all interrogativity. Me suddenly crying and crying.

"I can't bear the thought that you want this kid constantly haled out of her room, back into the space of the family, in the name of togetherness and mental hygiene. I think it's just plain true that I would not have survived. I really wouldn't."

"*Why?*"

"Because my main experience back then was of being submerged, over and over, in the most corrosive acid of anxiety. And if I hadn't had this solitude—and this resource for discharging, reconstituting myself—just for doing *something* . . . ! If I'd had *that* stripped away, and constantly got plunged back into the scene of it all . . . !"

I feel as if I'm describing a form of torture.

Shannon spends a while trying to get me to say why "it all" felt quite *that* way. I can't a bit—I'm naming the normal ebbs, flows, ragged edges of family and group dynamics; there's no one overarching exacerbation.

But it does seem as though some structure, some experiential quality of "back then," has arrived with an awful alacrity—a place to start

but not, I hope, to
pay a long visit. Gusty,
rain-lashed weather, here.

————

CONTINUES ON THE THEME OF THE ANXIETY ATTENDANT ON HER IN THE FAM-
ILY SPACE. MEMORIES OF BEING TEASED/RIDICULED ABOUT NOT BEING ABLE TO
TAKE A JOKE, BEING THIN SKINNED, ETC. SHE OFTEN DID NOT FEEL PART OF/
BELIEVE SHE WAS PART OF THE FAMILY, AND SO WAS OPEN TO ATTACK FROM
VARIOUS MEMBERS. SHE ACTUALLY WAS DIFFERENT IN SKIN FROM ALL OF THE
OTHERS IN THE FAMILY AND SO WHEN THEY WENT TO THE BEACH SUMMERS
SHE BOTH WAS THE OBJECT OF A LOT OF GREASING AND CREAMING AND CON-
CERN, AND ALSO ALWAYS BURNED. THE TACTILE SENSE OF PAIN AND THE UN-
HAPPINESS AND ALIENNESS ARE VIVID IN HER MEMORY. NOW, WHEN SHE GOES
TO THE BEACH, SHE STAYS IN DURING THE DAY AND ENJOYS THE EVENING
WALKS. UNCLEAR WHY HER PARENTS DID NOT STRUCTURE THINGS TO ACCOM-
MODATE HER DIFFERENCE.

————

PHONE CALL WAKES HER UP FROM THIS A.M.'S DREAMS——DREAM OF TRYING ON
CLOTHES AND NOTICING BY THE BLOOD RUNNING DOWN HER LEGS AND ON
THE CLOTHES THAT SHE IS MENSTRUATING. IT IS 4 YEARS SINCE SHE HAS (SUD-
DEN MENOPAUSE FROM CHEMOTHERAPY). AS SHE WAKES SHE IS REMINDED OF
A THOMAS MANN NOVELLA SHE DISLIKED, *THE BLACK SWAN*, IN WHICH AN
OLDER WOMAN FALLS IN LOVE AND BEGINS BLEEDING AGAIN, AT FIRST THINK-
ING THAT IT IS BECAUSE OF THE REAWAKENING OF HER PASSIONS, LATER TO
FIND OUT THAT IT IS UTERINE CANCER AND DIES. E BRINGS UP IMAGE OF HER
MOTHER AND W., AUTHENTIC DISCOVERIES AND PASSIONS OF LATER LIFE AS AN-
TIDOTE TO THIS VINDICTIVE PLOT.

———————

RE MENOPAUSE, TALKS ABOUT HOT FLASHES HAVING BROUGHT HER INTO THER-
APY IN THE FIRST PLACE——DRAMATIZING SHAME, HEAT, AFFECTIVE AURA OF
FEELING AWFUL AND "BAD"—— "MADE ME ABLE TO THINK ABOUT AFFECT AS A
TOPIC"——HAVING SEEN HERSELF AS SOMEONE WITHOUT EMOTIONS OR WITH-
OUT ACCESS TO THEM——WAS ABLE TO QUESTION THIS WHEN AFFECTS AND BOD-
ILY SENSATIONS CAME TO HER AS IF FROM OUTSIDE, AS A SYMPTOM, IN THE
FORM OF HOT FLASHES.

———————

QUIET WEEKEND. WENT TO BOOKSTORE IN NY AND FOUND COPY OF MICHAEL
BALINT, *BASIC FAULT*. TALKING ABOUT A WARM AND QUIET ENVIRONMENT AS
PART OF THERAPEUTIC TRANSFERENCE INSTEAD OF THE ANGER, SUSPICION,
MORTIFYING SELF-LOSS SHE HAD IMAGINED——REASSURED THAT WHAT WE ARE
DOING IS ON RIGHT TRACK.

   —Not in love with a
person—but with the place the
person inhabits

   and with the space of
my friendly distance from him.
Nor insatiable

but, in fact, content.
Nor demanding. Nor always
to be frustrated—

rather, to be pleased.
Grateful, trusting, yes, tender.
Happy, *therefore* good.

A GOOD LECTURE TRIP. REPORTS SOME POSITIVE FEELINGS AND SOME DECREASE
IN ANXIETY——DUE TO THE ZOLOFT?

About the decision to antidepress, finally, Shannon's all encouragement and interest—once I've made it. He's never made a move to
bring it closer. What I feel though is that, valuing my energy, he's
pleased with the lessened struggle to stay functional

and he enjoys my
habitable space—where the
floor is now higher.

5

I often, silently, try to guess how Shannon experiences his fatness—what he even calls it to himself—why he never so describes it, or chimes in with me on the subject—and whether he ever shares the depth of my rage and damage around fat issues. I wonder how, for him, his size may have intersected in ways I can't even imagine with activity, comfort, even authority.

And beyond the fatness. Which maybe seems small or accidental to him! I try to imagine

> a body in which
> motility is not the
> same thing as danger.

Maneuvering him into self-description, I learn he grew up un-athletic from a fat childhood; never acquired those masculine large-muscle skills; but he's deft and sure-footed. Feels secure going down stairs. Jumps from rock to rock on mountainsides. Knows his center of gravity intimately.

And I infer: a first child and a boy, he's never experienced his fatness as a totalizing matter of a ruined, sick, or offensive body.

> Some inches of him
> might be welcomed more warmly
> than other inches

but his whole, graceful
body is poised on knowing
how it *is* welcome.

———————

DREAM OF YOU AND A BUNCH OF YOUR OTHER PATIENTS, AND OTHER PEOPLE
—SOME KIND OF EXERCISE OR MEDICAL PROCEDURE INVOLVING DISCRETE LIT-
TLE HOPS—I BEGAN DANCING, DANCED OVER TO YOU AND YOU GOT DRAWN
INTO IT, VERY CLOSE TO ME, SOME IMPROPRIETY, BUT THE OTHERS HAD BEGUN
DANCING TOO . . .

———————

TELLS A DREAM THAT SHE HAD OF BEING ON A SUBMARINE WITH SOMEONE
WHO SHE FELT WAS ME. GOING DEEPER AND DEEPER IN SUBMARINE, BEING AL-
MOST HALF ASLEEP, FEELING GOOD. THEN HAVING A BABY WHICH IS "SO
HEALTHY THAT IT POKED ITS HEAD RIGHT OUT THROUGH THE PLACENTUM!"
SHE ASSOCIATES THE WORD ON WAKING AS PLEASANT TUM. SOMEHOW HARKING
BACK TO OUR TALKING ABOUT WEIGHT AND BODY SIZE.

I don't say so but
I know: this is *Shannon*'s round
and radiant tum.

———————

But then when we've gotten up to go after this session and we're con-
firming our times for the next week or two, suddenly I notice Shannon suspended motionless, gazing dumbly at his appointment book.
I wait, patient, for about half a minute. Then, "Yesss?" I quiz him.

He looks up with a strange smile.

"Well," he says, "I seem to have somebody else's name written
down for eleven next Friday. And it isn't that I got mixed up and made
an appointment with somebody else, either—I knew it was with you.
I just wrote down somebody else's name instead."

There's a long, odd silence. I feel vastly amused, I guess at the "psychoanalytic" stylization of this moment. Also funnily touched. Also I suppose ready to feel insulted (who's been eating my porridge?), though not actually feeling so. Want to say something

> like, well, sweetheart, *you're*
> the shrink, you're supposed to tell
> me what all this means.

But Shannon remains very taken aback—for him it's too early to laugh. I see there's something disproportionate going on, but I've no way of knowing whether it's *all* about me, his feelings for me, or *none*. Or just a little. Is this a joke I'm in on, that I make the pith of—or is there some other intimacy on his docket, so vastly stronger or sweeter than ours that even to associate the two makes a joke?

It feels unexpectedly haimish and familiar, this included/excluded relation to Shannon's inner process.

I'm also noting, the discussion of slips of this kind has formed no part of our discourse. I'd looked forward to it in advance, but I've only had reason to feel how resistant he always seems to focusing on the level of the signifier. Yet this mistake really captures him—captures and throws him.

Finally I can gather my wits a little and say, I hope affectionately and lightly (but I'm not sure), "I guess if you really want to see someone else during that hour, it could be arranged."

To which he responds with, again, disproportionate amusement or *something*: still with the appointment book open at his waist, he swings back on his heels in a 360-degree revolution of inarticulacy to wind up facing me again, laughing heartily—and we say a cheerful goodbye.

Odd little man.

————

This year I'm doing an insane amount of lecture travel. Week after week. I feel the cost of it one morning sitting in an airplane on the runway in Toronto. Anti-icing fluid (with which the plane is being sluiced) suddenly running pink down the window beside me, looking like Pepto-Bismol, but it comes on my sight like horror: what I am seeing, I think, is (something I hadn't thought of from that day to this) the bloody discharge from tubes in the week or so after the surgery.

Yes, as a matter of fact, it is the anniversary of my diagnosis.

I'm learning that "I've been abandoned" is easier for me to feel than "I am afraid."

Another lecture trip gets off to an upsetting start: an old woman in one of those airline wheelchairs is rolled to a seat a good ways behind me. But something must have happened in her transfer to the airplane seat: the plane is soon permeated with miserable weeping she can't seem to stop. (At least, I assume it's she. I actually can't see.)

This is upsetting. I helplessly identify with her weeping; I'm plunged into an incident where I was ignored for a couple of hours in the hospital, waiting for surgery to implant an IV port in my arm for chemo. I was naked, flat on my back, under a sheet on a gurney—tears coursing wretchedly into my *ears*—and couldn't get the attention of the horrid nurses who were supposed to be minding the empty pre-op room. This was about a month after the mastectomy, which I'd sailed through in high spirits and *bon courage*; probably I was unexpectedly brought face to face with a lot of fear from that experience that now, when my guard was down and my denial less mobilized, was able to ambush me.

Yet my fear of the coming operation, if it was fear, still didn't register as fear but as a disconsolate sense that I already *had been abandoned*. And that

> I *was* abandoned,
> in the sense that there was no
> controlling that grief,

that outrage. A crazy regression, an infantile compulsion. But maybe an alternative to looking forward with dread?

———

WEIRD, PUNISHING DREAMS—FASCIST TAKEOVER BY THE FACULTY COMMITTEE ORGANIZED TO CHOOSE THE ANGLICAN MARTYR FOR THE ANNUAL CELEBRATION. SCARED. KNEW THAT THEY WOULD COME TO ROUND UP AND KILL HER CAT—HOW TO GET IT TO THE SAFETY OF THE HOSPITAL ACROSS THE PARTIALLY FROZEN LAKE? WEIGHS TOO MUCH BUT CAN GO OUT TILL THE ICE STARTS BREAKING, THEN HEAD BACK TOWARD THE SHORE, BREAKING OFF ICE, UNTIL SHE CAN WADE AROUND THE EDGE OF THE LAKE AGAINST THE BROKEN EDGES, CARRYING THE CAT TO THE HOSPITAL. COMING BACK HOME, HEARING THUNDERING NOISES OF CANNONS AND GUNS—SCARED. SECOND DREAM—NOTICES POWDERED BLOOD IN TOILET AND UNDERPANTS—CONCLUDES SHE WAS RAPED AND NEEDS TO GO TO DOCTOR. IT'S SNOWING—PUSHING HER CAR THERE— DOCTOR IS LEAVING—CATCHES HIM OUTSIDE—HIS SENSE THAT THE BLOOD HAD BEEN TAMPED INSIDE HER BY A PENIS, BUT SENSE ALSO THAT IT WAS HER PENIS—WAKES FEELING STRESSED, TIRED, BURDENED. THOUGHTS—GOTTA GET MY PUSSY SOMEWHERE—ATMOSPHERE OF UNDEFINED THREAT AND COLD—

———

Another scare about a possible cancer symptom—this one, grotesquely, a foot pain.

We try to trace it back and back, the whirlpool of panic, guilt, and fantasy, but however far into childhood I manage to take it, it's always the same. Somehow there has always been something I needed from symptoms or from illness (escape, attention, narrative substance, transport?) that would hijack and confound the simpler motive provided by the wish to have my pain relieved or to be healthy.

I've never known what I was supposed to ask of my pain.

But I get to remember the first time I ever fainted, when I was seven, at Nanny's house, where I'd been reading *Pinocchio*—reading about the fairy with azure hair. I'd no idea what azure was, but what a word.

    I knocked my funnybone somehow against a doorjamb—and

then I was waking
on the floor, where at first it
seemed quite natural

that people would be
saying, and with tenderness,
"Eve," and me with my

headful of azure—
    then disorientation—
then the whole rupture

of consciousness kind
of reconstructing itself—
backward. By magic.

———

BLUNT, CONTENTLESS, PHYSICAL ANXIETY LAST NIGHT ABOUT THE POSSIBILITY OF CANCER RECURRENCE—SHOULD SHE BE DOING SOMETHING ABOUT IT BEFORE UPCOMING TRIPS? CAN THE USUAL DEFENSES KICK IN? ANXIETY IS ABOUT BEING SICK FOR A LONG TIME WHICH A RECURRENCE WOULD REPRESENT. — ISOLATION OF MORTALITY ISSUES AND FEELINGS, ESTRANGEMENT FROM THE FEELINGS ABOUT IT—SIMILAR TO THE PRIOR ESTRANGEMENT FROM FEELINGS OF SEXUALITY.— "OH, HERE'S A COMFORTING THOUGHT; I MIGHT HAVE AN INCURABLE ILLNESS" BUT THEN IT'S NOT A COMFORTING THOUGHT, BUT I STILL ORGANIZE SO MUCH OF MY ENERGY, THINKING, ETC., AROUND THAT. HABITUALLY, IT OFTEN IS ODDLY COMFORTING, LIKE GRABBING ONTO YOUR CROTCH FOR REASSURANCE. IT'S LIKE THERE ARE PLACES INSIDE ME WHERE EVERYTHING'S REVERSED.

———

Nice therapy moment: Shannon asks, Is there anything you'd like me to *do* about all this anxiety you're experiencing?

Me (saying this at exactly the moment that Shannon realizes it is what I am about to say and that he has no answer to this question): What did you have in mind?

Shannon

(perhaps wildly): Oh—
pat you on the head? Tell you
it'll be all right?

Me: Oh, I'm taking that as done.

PROBLEM WITH PAIN PROBABLY NOT MALIGNANT, BIOPSY RESULTS BACK TUES. FEELING AN EXIT CLOSED OFF, EXIT FROM WORLD WHICH IS TERRIBLE AND GETTING WORSE, AND FROM HAVING TO BE HERSELF. SELF—SWIRLING GRAY LOST CONFUSED BORING NOTHINGNESS PARTLY ABOUT JUST BEING ME AND PARTLY ABOUT THERAPY. WHEN WE ARE MESHING I'M HAPPY, A WHILE SINCE I'VE FELT LIKE THAT. A RECURRENCE WOULD HAVE GIVEN AN UNDERLYING NARRATIVE CONSISTENCY, FOCUS, RATIONALE FOR OUR TASK. ASKS IF I THINK IT'S TIME TO TURN AND WALK AWAY OR DOES IT CLEAR A SPACE FOR US TO WORK? (NOT A, B) WHY NOT A? (WOULD BE HARD NOT TO SEE YOU, DOESN'T FEEL RIGHT INTUITIVELY, POSED ISSUES ESP. ABOUT SEXUALITY THAT WE HAVE LEFT UNATTENDED.) OK, BUT I SEEM TO NOT HAVE GOTTEN OVER THE SENSE THAT ONE HAS TO BE VERY SICK TO DESERVE THIS KIND OF ATTENTION. I'M NOT PHYSICALLY SICK AND DON'T FEEL EMOTIONALLY SICK NOWADAYS. ALSO IT'S AWFUL TO THINK OF GIVING UP THE NARRATIVE SPACE OF THERAPY.—TRANSFERENTIAL STUFF—I'VE ALWAYS ASSUMED THAT WE WOULD BE FRIENDS AFTER THERAPY— THE RECURRENCE NARRATIVE WOULD MAKE WHAT WE DO WITH EACH OTHER SIMPLE AND UNPROBLEMATIC, E.G., I COULD HAVE YOU HOLD MY HAND AND I WOULDN'T BE UPSET BY THAT.

Back, this time, from a lecture trip to California. Where my best, and most worrying, visit has been with Gary Fisher, a former student. Gary is a quicksilver young black writer who won't show his ravishing stories and won't tell anyone—won't let me tell anyone—about the HIV that is working its way through his incandescent body.

He's been healthy so far. So far as I know, anyhow, he has.

But all through this visit, a horrible cough is shuddering behind his light voice. Asthma, he says.

I tell Shannon I've fallen in deep again with Gary; more practically, that I've finally succeeded in raising the topic of money with him; I'm relieved that he has let me do so.

At the moment, I'm glad I already know that Shannon takes care of people himself. He's told me he has a niece and nephew living with him along with a kid and stepkid; he seems to have the adopting habit. My assuming this responsibility won't alarm him.

All he says is, You
realize you're in for the
duration?
    I do.

What seems true is that I've somehow, in the last few weeks, gotten terrified. The best description I can give Shannon: I've lost my third dimension. I have the sensation that the front and back of my chest cavity are glued together with fear; there's no place for my hammering heart, no interiority. No rooms to go into, and no one to go into them. I'm so much at bay that my whole materiality has flattened.

And I have to go on the road again: a lecture at Notre Dame tomorrow.

Shannon says, I see you *pushing against*—something, someone.

Pushing against him, in particular, he says; he sees him and me pushing against each other.

"Pushing against"—it takes me several beats to realize he means this literally. It is a suggestion of something that might happen. It's not his image of, say, how his and my conversations may have gotten me into this pickle in the first place.

He returns to the topic and I remember our recent goodbye, where he mentioned patting me on the head and I cleverly said I would take the act as done. Suddenly it comes over me that he heard that as a refusal of a proffer, and I realize after that, it could only be because he had in mind that he might have literally patted me on the head.

(Which I think I would have liked. But I certainly assumed the rules were that my shrink and I could not touch.)

So, no, he is saying that it might wake me up from this bad-dream feeling a little if I can get up and push against someone—him, or (as I don't make a response) Michael when I get home, if Michael would do something like that; or just to think about it, if that's what I would feel comfortable with . . .

I think I am rather shocked with this. I'm sure I am. But at once it seems that, having arrived with instantaneous suddenness at this dangerous threshold, I will have to cross now and look back at it later. If I "just think about it" or do it at home with Mike, it will only supercharge the site of a physical contact that will, in any event, no longer be able to present itself to me as out of bounds.

Once it comes to me,
so strangely, that he means it—
I guess it's happened.

So up rise I, in lieu of answer; and up rises Shannon. And planting our feet and ourselves about a yard apart, we place hand against hand, his and mine, and push with our little might to force each other a step or two backward.

I've begun with no idea what to expect: will he be far bigger and stronger than I? Will I be far bigger and stronger than he? With each other we've been so disembodied.

In fact we prove to be the same height and pretty evenly matched. We push for a while without either of us getting anywhere. Step back from each other, panting ostentatiously, though clearly we've been pulling our punches.

I move to join again. And having somehow recovered my concentration, and realizing that in order

> to push him backward
> I'll have to be ready to
> move forward on him,

I do so and actually succeed in budging him a little.

Whereupon, back to his chair, my couch, the footstool that we always share, our feet delicately poised at its opposite corners.

And how do I feel now?

For starters, I immediately *do* feel better,

> embodied in quite
> a new way; dimensional,
> powerful.
>> *Not scared,*

so that was a good intuition that Shannon had.

Then, of course, I am disquieted at this tectonic shift in what I've presumed were the fixed zones of permission and prohibition.

Also, though, I feel somehow restored to an adult size—in relation, that is, to the spectral figure of my fear and rage. Which I've always associated with my father in his own rage: a figure who's abstract to me in the particular sense that it could never have occurred to me to resist or push back against him, or to wrestle him to a standstill or to anything else.

My ambivalence.
After the session, Shannon
writes down his home phone

number on his card—I'm supposed to call from the Midwest if I feel awful again this weekend. I put it in my pocket and sort of forget about it.

Getting home an hour or two later, I reach into my pocket, happy to find his card there. What a comforting thing to have and hold. I take it out and look at his round handwriting with pleasure, then put it back in my pocket. Immediately I think: gee, these pants are dirty; since I'm leaving for Notre Dame at seven A.M., if I'm going to wash them it had better be right this minute.

It isn't for half an hour that I picture them tumbling around the washer and realize . . .

"A true fact I keep reminding myself to tell you—though I suppose you might have guessed.

"It's that—though of course I'm an atheist, bone and sinew—the belief in hell is powerful in me."

I don't know why. It hardly runs in the family.

I think I've read that, among Christians, something like ninety-seven percent are confident of being bound for heaven. What unimaginable fatuity!

Maybe it's from my dreams that I know about hell. The recurrent ones where the premise of the dream is to recognize that I've done something—killed someone—and while I can't remember the event, or it seemed small at the time, nothing, nothing ever can undo it.

Too late the Gothic
bellstroke tumbling and tumbling
over these dread dreams—

too late in knowing, that is, or too late in making the act real to myself. Too late ever again to make it different. The danger was my distraction, forgetfulness, casual brutality, my desire to please, or absence of mind.

Always, the waking from such dreams: a heaven of new possibility, of relief.

————

Were one not to wake!
Were there to be no other
world into which to.

————

It's a Nietzschean hell, I suppose, a hell of unrefreshment. Shannon is wondering how it relates to that other of my groundtones: the longing for death. Which I wonder, too.

It's not necessarily posthumous, for one thing. It could as easily happen in this life. It's why I've always known I couldn't have an abortion ("though I'll defend to the death your right" et cetera). Suppose I talked myself into its being just fine—and then someday the floor of knowing that simply dropped away for good. Or, I mean, some stark light supervened, a shriveling light in which . . .

Depression is probably another name for that bony light?

Or depression, a name for the swale where nothing can turn out differently?

Here is a graphic image of hell for me. When I taught outside Utica, I had two cats, sisters, Harpo and Beishung, whom I'd adopted as kittens. As kittens they enjoyed and amused each other, but then as they got older they fought constantly. And one of them, Harpo, turned out to be impossible to love—for me, anyway. It was as if she didn't know how to be made happy.

She was a nice kitty, beautiful, with long, irresistibly soft black fur. She looked plump and full, but if you ever saw her wet you saw a pitiful rat. And she did hunger: for love, for attention. Her nose was always in your armpit, her paws on your paper, her butt straining up from your lap into your touch. And she was a machine for purring—loud, insistent, wanting.

Yet, somehow what she wanted wasn't ever what she wanted. The moment of contentment, when the straining subsides, purring smooths to a barely audible snore,

> tissues dissolve in
> a heavy, companionate
> mercury puddle

like her sister's—such moments for her never would seem to arrive.

So it was clear to me I'd have to get rid of one of the cats and that Harpo was the one. I was too ashamed to take her to the SPCA—what reason could I give them? She has a personality disorder? She won't cuddle? She reminds me of my mother-in-law?

I'd heard enough about the scandalous cruelty of abandoning cats to know that abandoning cats is something people often do.

So I put her into her carrier in the car and drove out of town, west along a ridge of mountains. It was March, and for a wonder not too snowy. The ground was bald and hard, bitten away like bark, and sharp with stony outcrops. I'd never driven this route before.

When we were high up, we came to a small, battered graveyard by the side of the road. With quick decision I stopped the car; climbed out; and pulled out the carrier in which she'd been cowering, quiet and carsick, curled up small. Unlatching the top of it, I laid it down and waited for her to step out.

My fantasy had been that she'd bound away in terror from me, the car, and her carrier, I suppose—terror at the ominous ride, the strange menace of the scene. She would bound away and I, unable to pursue her, would drive off. But that course of action didn't seem to cross her so-called mind. She was slow in stepping out of the carrier—slow enough for me to feel the tooth of a wind that set about to gnaw through my own coat. Once she'd unfolded her inky skeins, even, she barely ventured. All dainty, and frightened she stood her ground within inches of the carrier, damp black nose tasting the air, and seemingly felt no reason to move any farther from shelter. Clearly, there was a bitter storm on the way. Its clouds sent shadows gadding over us as we stood there, making me small, her tiny. She was very still, only beginning to shiver with the raveling of her black rags.

So that was how I knew hell. It was clear to me that if I left her there alone, I'd find myself just there like that, just as alone and forever, at some arbitrary moment in the future dead or living. Or else, that the place of that moment would suddenly sometime recur, in all its immediacy and hate, inside me, for good.

This knowledge of hell was very tied to the particular place.

So I took Harpo back in the car with me and we found our way to the SPCA. "I have to move to an apartment that doesn't allow cats," I brazened, and left her there to find whatever fate she'd encounter.

Oddly, it felt okay to leave her there—it didn't trigger any punishing superstition.

———

ANOTHER DREAM ABOUT ME IN WHICH SHE ASKS ME IF I HAVE BEEN SOMEWHAT MUTED LATELY, AND IN THE DREAM I TELL HER YES, I HAVE BEEN DEPRESSED. I SAY THERE IS SOME ACCURACY IN THE DREAM AS I HAVE BEEN MUTED/DEPRESSED. BESIDES THIS E REFLECTS ON HER RESPONSE WHEN I SEEM DEPRESSED AS IT MAY REFLECT HOW SHE RESPONDED TO HER MOTHER'S POSSIBLE DEPRESSION AFTER HER BIRTH AND THE STILLBIRTH BEFORE HER BROTHER WAS BORN. SHE NOTES THAT SHE MUTES SOME HERSELF, GRAYS OUT HER NEEDS AND AFFECT, SOME IN THE SERVICE OF A JOINING/MERGING WITH THE DEPRESSED PERSON, THEN TRYING TO INJECT SOME LIFE INTO THE CORD OF THE RELATIONSHIP. CAN FEEL HERSELF DOING THIS WITH ME.

———

REACTING TO MY SAYING I WAS DEPRESSED. WOKE UP MON NIGHT IN FRIGHT —PARTLY THAT SHE HAD HAD A BAD CLASS MON (CAN'T TEACH OR PERFORM

RIGHT), PARTLY THAT SHE WAS AFRAID OF LOSING ME OR SOMETHING OF ME
INTO A DEPRESSION. "I CAN'T TELL THE DIFFERENCE BETWEEN SOMEONE I LOVE
BEING DEPRESSED VS. SUICIDAL." HER OWN SUICIDAL IDEATION MAKES SUCH
IMAGES IMPINGE VERY CLOSE ON HER. ASKS ABOUT HOW DO I THINK I AM AND
WHAT MY EXPERIENCE OF DEPRESSION IS. REALIZES THAT THIS TAPS SOME OLD
INTERACTION WITH HER MOTHER.

"When you say you're depressed—well, would you describe yourself
as *pretty* depressed, or *just a little bit* depressed, or . . . well, quite depressed?"

He laughs, trying to think about it. Finally says, "I can tell you
more substantively what it feels like for me. When I get depressed my
image for it, at its worst, is being a prehistoric man, shut up in a cave,
everything gray and cold, with just one fire and, say, one rock. For me
it's mostly about withdrawal, about losing interest—you know how
usually I'm interested in everything. So it's striking when I'm not.

"But then, in this imagery I seem to have developed long ago, as
soon as I'm a little better, it's as though there's a short walk I can take,
away downhill somewhere from the cave, and there's a little lake
there, and some rocks by the side of it. So I can sit still on one of the
rocks and look into the lake. That's about how it's been for me lately."

I'm worried that there's something volatile going on in his head,
scared of his going into a tailspin or something if the wrong chord
gets plucked.

"Nah, I don't think so. For me it's mainly boring—I'm impatient
for it to get over with. No, it's a long time since I've had the sense of
being depressed enough to get scared by it."

E WORRIES, DID I FIND HER QUESTIONS LAST TIME INTRUSIVE RE MY DEPRES-
SION? BUT I TELL HER NO, I FEEL SEEN BY HER AND THAT THAT IS AN ENCOUR-
AGEMENT.

We stumble back to a notation that really struck me as right.

Namely: I envision my bond with my mother as a therapy relationship, in which I am the therapist. Probably I have always related to her in this way.

> That is: I've had an
> immemorial motive
> of eliciting,
>
> supporting, helping
> *her* inhabit and extend
> a certain "true self"

rather than a more available false self, that nursery school "mother."

Shannon likes the idea. But he wants me to feel, too, the important difference from real therapy: that this therapist *needed* and yearned for exposure to that true self of the patient's.

(Maybe all that made it "true" was that it *was* what I needed?)

> It comes to me, too,
> that even though it was my
> own, childish needs that
>
> drove the "therapy,"
> our practice must also have
> required me (or else—
>
> permitted me?) to
> learn a rather imposing
> habit of silence
>
> about my own needs.
> Hasn't that been *the* major
> defense I've mounted

against my mother
all these years?—defense of *and*
also against her.

———————

THIS TURNED INTO A VERY UNUSUAL SESSION. BEGAN WITH REPORTING ON
LECTURES IN QUEBEC. SHE SAYS SHE HAD BEEN FEELING AN IMPATIENCE VIS-À-
VIS THERAPY LATELY AND A MIASMIC MOOD AROUND HER THAT HAD CRYSTAL-
LIZED INTO THE IMPATIENCE. ASKED WHAT MY EXPERIENCE HAD BEEN——I SAY
MORE POSITIVE IN THAT I HAD SEEN HER FOCUSING ON THE TRANSFERENTIAL
ASPECTS MORE. I ASKED SOMEWHERE IN HERE IF THERE WAS SOME ANGER IN
THE IMPATIENCE OR IN SOMETHING AND SHE AGREED——I ASKED IF THAT
ANGER WAS SOMETHING SHE COULD RECALL FROM CHILDHOOD——SHE DOES
NOT RESONATE TO THAT ALTHOUGH SHE SAYS SHE BELIEVES IT MUST HAVE BEEN
THERE. I SAY SOMETHING ABOUT ITS BEING REPRESSED OR SUPPRESSED A LOT.

ANOTHER UNCLEAR TRANSITION BUT WITH HER BEGINNING TO TALK ABOUT
HOW IT HAS SEEMED TO HER THAT I HAVE BEEN SEEING HER AS VERY CON-
STRICTED, HEDGED ABOUT, AND INEXPRESSIVE OF HERSELF. AS THIS LINE CON-
TINUES SHE IS INCREASINGLY DISTRAUGHT AT IDEA THAT I SEE HER AS
"PALLID," WHICH IS A WAY SHE SAYS NO ONE ELSE SEES HER AND SHE NEVER
SEES HERSELF. SHE FEELS INSTEAD THAT SHE WAS DEMONIC, POWERFUL, AND
UNIQUE (IN AN ANOMALOUS SENSE). IS VERY UPSET THAT SHE THINKS I HAVE
COMPLETELY MISSED THIS IN HER AND THAT HER ENTIRE UNDERSTANDING OF
HERSELF HAS BEEN MISSED AND THUS UNDONE BY ME. WE GO ROUND AND
ROUND ON THIS FOR A WHILE——MY TRYING DEFENSIVELY TO CLARIFY AND EX-
PLAIN (I HAVE BEEN SEEING THE WEAKER, OPPRESSED, HAPLESS OR HELPLESS
ASPECT OF HER OR HER SITUATION FOR A WHILE——FOCUSING ON YOUNGER
YEARS EVEN WHEN SHE HAS TALKED OF OLDER YEARS).

I FEEL LIKE I WAS PUSHED INTO A POSITION VIS-À-VIS HER THAT WAS NOT MINE
AND WAS TRYING TO EXPLAIN MY WAY OUT OF IT. I AM NOT SURE IF I HAVE
BEEN RESPONDING TO HER WRONGLY AND SHE IS UPBRAIDING ME FOR IT, OR
IF SHE IS PROJECTING ONTO ME ATTITUDES SHE EXPERIENCED FROM PARENTS
REGARDING HER INTELLIGENCE, AGGRESSIVENESS, ETC., OR IF THIS IS A RE-

SPONSE TO THE RECENT TOPIC OF HER RAGE IN CHILDHOOD, OR WHAT?? I SAY I
AM SURE I HAVE NOT MISSED HER DEMONIC QUALITY BUT THAT I HAVE NOT
FELT IT IN THE WAY HER PARENTS DID—PARTLY AS I'M NOT HER PARENTS,
PARTLY AS MY PARENTS RESPONDED TO THIS SORT OF THING DIFFERENTLY. THIS
SEEMS TRANSFERENTIAL MUDDLE AND I NEED SOME PERSPECTIVE ON IT. WE
WENT ABOUT 1-1/2 HRS AND FOR THE FIRST TIME I HUGGED HER AT THE
END—AN IMPULSE I'VE HAD BEFORE BUT ONLY NOW ACTED ON, PROBABLY OUT
OF WANTING NOT TO HAVE HURT HER AS SHE FEELS HURT, PARTLY TO TRY TO
RECONNECT, PARTLY OUT OF MY OWN BEING VERY SHAKEN BY THE INTENSITY
OF THE CONFLICT BETWEEN US.??

Afterward it comes back only in disconnected bits, which I then can't
remember—trying to round up in my mind—a bit like trauma, "stop-
less, cool."

One pattern of this fight: I keep insisting that anyone who knew
anything about me at all could not help but perceive me as "a wild animal," demonic, uncanny, suffering, and sui generis. (Anything but
pallid, in short.) He keeps insisting that I did not have to be those
things. "When I think of you as a child I see someone very bright, very
creative, interesting, really *nice* . . ."

Which is about the nadir of the thing.

Me: "I feel as though suddenly I'm being turned into a middle
child again."

It all makes me feel how strong my family romance fantasies are.
Like, You don't understand, you can't understand, I'm *exceptional*, my
parents are the emperor and empress of Mars. How can I possibly
prove it to you? How can you possibly not already know it?

Latish in the conversation he says to me, "Well, you've certainly
gotten my attention."

I respond coolly,
"As you know, that is the height
of my ambition."

It's interesting, at the beginning of the next hour, trying to put our stories together. He says that like me, he's tried and tried to piece it together, what on earth happened, and been unable to. "These snatches of conversation would keep coming into my head," he says, "but I had no idea how we'd gotten from one to another. Where did all this come from?"

He laughs out loud when I tell him the translation Tim offered for his adjective "pallid": "shy and doesn't have a great tan."

He asks whether some of this melodrama was a necessary/difficult way of telling him he isn't treating me right. I say I don't know, but one set of issues that's gotten very stirred up for me in the last week is about his (yes, I use this word) complacency.

I say as long as I can remember, with him, I've had these two streams of feeling. One, that it's very reassuring, relaxing, enabling to me that he seems so relaxed about who and how he is. He's so undefensive and unthreatened, *unbrittle*—so promisingly different from (say) my parents.

But then, I can also see him as maddeningly complacent—in the ways I'm prone to associate with straight male presumption.

"Can you say more," Shannon wonders, "what you mean, 'complacent'?"

I try out a few formulations and settle on: "You acted as though *you* had nothing at stake."

It's all involved with my surmises about what our therapy feels like to him. What I've liked to think, and often have been able to, is that somehow he does put more at risk with me than usual with his patients. That maybe I manage to stretch the boundaries, somehow, of what he thinks he knows—of what he knows he can already do.

I say, "It's meant a lot to me to imagine the therapy as an adventure or experiment for you—not just me.

"But," I add, anticipating a kind letdown, "I guess your best answer would be that that happens for you, one way or another, in every therapy?"

He furrows a brow at me. "This is one of those times when I feel torn: I think it would be really interesting to answer your question, *but*

I want to know more about your asking of it." Well, I say, I'd like an answer first.

"Okay, then, let me be truthful: sometimes it feels like that with you and sometimes it doesn't. But it's certainly truer in this therapy than in my other ones, at least right now.

"Somewhere early on with you, I threw away a set of routines that, with a lot of other patients, are almost all of what needs doing. You know: tell me more about that ... yes ... yes ... and this started when? That's what it takes with many people—it's pretty boring for me, though, except insofar as it's like playing with a chemistry set.

"Whereas I do feel as though what you and I are up to is an experiment, yes, and an adventure. I feel as though I'm *here* in it in a way I'm not a lot of the time. Of course I like that.

"But then sometimes I remember in a scary way that what happens to you is going to depend in some real sense on what I'm like. And then I think: what if I'm wrong? I mean not as in right or wrong, not as in doing or saying the wrong thing, but just—wrong. In my way of being. So, yeah, there is the sense of being at stake in all this in a different way than the usual.

"Of course a lot of the time I do try to make myself scarce, back off, leave plenty of space between us to see what you'll fill it with."

At the very end of the hour he asks if there's anything he or I should say about the hug he gave me. And I say no, I was grateful he did it.

Especially because our words, our thoughts, were so angry, it was crucial to know that

> still somewhere else—in
> our two bodies—our bond did
> stubbornly subsist.

ENTIRE STORM GONE. A LIGHT SESSION. NOW IT IS HARD TO FULLY REMEMBER WHAT SHE WAS DOING THIS FOR. I ASK @ CHILDHOOD FIGHTS ESPECIALLY THEIR AFTERMATH—SHE WOULD GO OFF BY HERSELF AND CRY UNTIL SHE

COULD ACT CALMER BUT STILL FELT VERY TURBULENT AND THEN RETURN TO
TALK W/ PARENTS. IN THE INCIDENTS SHE CAN REMEMBER, SHE WOULD
QUICKLY ESCALATE ISSUE TO A WIN/LOSE, LIFE/DEATH LEVEL.

I'm saying to him, "Pallid or not, I suppose it's true I see myself as
quite a timid person—though also, I guess, courageous, in a different
register. But maybe you see me as timid in ways I don't even have a
clue about."

And he nods seriously.

But he adds: "I don't think timidity is just a trait that lives inside a
person, but instead, something relational.

"There are lots of things that are perfectly easy if you're doing them
with someone else, but almost impossible if you feel you're doing
them alone."

> Which is just plain true!
> Like going to a party
> where no one knows you—
>
> excruciating
> by yourself, effortless when
> a friend will come too—

And at once it's vivid to me again, the bliss of moving within a beloved
aegis.

It feels more than protective. It feels electrifying.

> The pride, in childhood,
> of going anywhere with
> my older sister!
>
> The extravagant
> rightness of it! Intimate
> sanction for us two,

to be sealed with my
favorite pronoun: the dear
first person plural.

It never surprised *me* that "we," in French, means yes.

Even in adulthood I'm addicted to the word. "Oh, yes, we saw that movie." "Our favorite restaurant." "We figured out—"

Hal, Michael, my family, students, friends, find it puzzling. "*We* saw that? Not that I remember."

Secretly this is a matter of pride to me.

Promiscuous we!
Me, plus anybody else.
Permeable we!

6

I want to know, "Don't you ever find yourself suspicious when I'm so sanguine about these intimate relationships—Hal, Michael, friends, students? Don't you wonder, can that much good relating really happen? And where are all the conflicts?"

With some thought, he says, "For a long time I was aware of staying agnostic about it. Not suspicious, but close to that. But over time, I guess I've figured that if you've been systematically misperceiving all these relationships—well, it is systematic; it seems to work in a consistent way for you.

"But also, over time, I can see from our interactions how you *are* good at intimacy."

"—and terrible at conflict!" I add.

"Well, y-yeah. But then I can picture these relationships better, and they make sense enough. It's not as though you never talk about conflicts, either—so when they come up so rarely it makes me think either they *are* rare, or anyway they're not looming too large for you—

"Are you asking this because you want to flash me a yellow light?"

"No, no, I don't think so. But I sometimes wonder

whether you think I
overidealize my
friends. Kind of wholesale."

"You think?"

"I think about it, sure. Last week Mary described me to myself as 'scattering sequins over us all'—all the people I love. She's right, she and they do seem so glamorous and numinous to me. I always see the light shaking out of their wings. It does shock me when anyone views them in an ordinary light—or worse, when they see each other that way."

Shannon says, "You don't seem so given to *dis*enchantment."

"Only with you!" I have to answer him laughing. "I seem to play that game over and over with you. My Barbie doll to dress and undress.

"Otherwise, really no. Except for very early in relationships. It's as though I want to start out powdering people with fairy dust when I first know them—like there's a working hypothesis that I'll trust them, we're playing the same exciting game, that they're radiant, kind, mysteriously talented, spiritually powerful. With lots of people the sequins naturally drop off soon, quite without melodrama or, really, embitterment. But if people stay numinous to me for a while, then there they are—in the pantheon.

"I guess it's very silly. At least, it's transparently narcissistic. Catering to my amour propre *is* a sure path to godhead. And threatening it . . . !"

Shannon says, yes, he does see me very given to such idealizations.

There's a long silence.

Often it's sobering to be agreed with.

———

I pick up with the idealizing habit, how it's related to being so depressive. Asking Shannon, "Do you think it's just defending me against a fearful certainty that, if I ever took off my emerald glasses, or stopped hurling sequins, the world around me would be exposed as black-and-white instead of in color; or awful; or just plain dead?"

Meaning: is all this
Bob Mackie glamour holding
on to one big lie?

"I see that sometimes that's exactly the feeling," Shannon says. "I've known other people besides you who do this, too. But actually it seems like a pretty wonderful adaptation.

"It makes them happier, and it makes the people around them different and better. It improves the environment."

"You mean it's *nice*."

"Well, yeah. Not *just* nice. But can you keep it in your head how very nice it is, and also that it's a kind of depressive idealization—at the same time?"

"You mean without ontologically ranking the two views of it?"

"Mm-hmm. Because it's the pressure to rank them that's *really* depressive, isn't it?"

———

MY WAY OF PAYING ATTENTION TO PEOPLE IS ADDITIVE, NON-NARRATIVE. THUS I DON'T HAVE A SENSE OF CHANGE IN PEOPLE, I.E., IF I NOTICE SOMETHING NEW I DON'T THINK "THEY'VE CHANGED." INSTEAD, I THINK, "THIS IS AN ADDITIONAL WAY X IS" — GROWS OUT OF SOME KIND OF STRESS ON OBJECT PERMANENCE, HOW TO KEEP THE SAME PERSON, A KIND OF CUBIST THREE-DIMENSIONALITY.

Yes, it makes persons my favorite study; makes them, to my taste, lovably, endlessly broodable-on.

Maybe it comes of having a changeable mother. Or one who's such a lover of "nuance."

With the view from outside, with the anxious view of a daughter, I see her oddly static. As though the love of paradox were her way of wrestling reality to a standstill? Except for overwhelming things, the body-blows of Nina's abandonment and, maybe, my cancer—

and the new love of
W., letting her play
the daughter—again—

but in her newfound mode, the key of sensuousness.

———————

AT THE END OF THE HOUR SHE SKETCHES A DREAM. SHE IS 10 MINUTES LATE
FOR AN APPOINTMENT WITH ME AND ARRIVES AT MY HOUSE, WHERE EVERY-
THING IS IN DISARRAY. I AM THERE, A NUMBER OF KIDS WHO KEEP POPPING
UP, PEOPLE COMING AND GOING, MY WIFE. E IS INCLUDED IN WHAT IS GOING
ON, BUT IS NOT ABLE TO GET MY FULL ATTENTION, ALTHOUGH HER FEELING IS
ALSO ONE OF INTIMACY AND PLEASURE. THERE IS A CHILD WHO IS BEING CARED
FOR BY A SEEMINGLY RETARDED WOMAN READING TO HIM. KID'S NAME IS
DAVID. E WAS LATE BECAUSE SHE HAD TROUBLE GETTING DRESSED, AND HER
CLOTHES ARE ON HER BODY IN SOMETHING OF A STUCK-ON MANNER. SHE HAS
BROUGHT A CHIFFON PIE AND NOTICES THAT HER BRA HAS GOTTEN BAKED
INTO A LAYER OF THE PIE. SHE PULLS IT OUT SAYING THAT SOME SCARF HAS
GOTTEN IN HERE, TRYING TO CONCEAL THAT IT IS HER BRA. I GO OFF INTO A
BATHROOM. SHE FINDS HERSELF UNDER A LAP ROBE WITH ANOTHER PERSON
AND MY WIFE, ARMS AROUND ONE ANOTHER'S SHOULDERS. SHE ASKS ABOUT
THE KIDS AND MY WIFE SAYS DAVID IS OUR SHADOW CHILD, AN EXPERIMENT
THAT FAILED. SHE REFLECTS ON HAVING COME TO SEE ME BUT ENDING UP
CLOSE WITH MY WIFE.

———————

Sessions that seem to yield—I don't know how to say it besides Something to chew on, or Something to hold on to—except that Something
to suck on is even truer. It's not so much thinking *more* about anything, as just the friendly, literal happiness that there's a flavor of an
exchange or two (maybe trapped between my teeth)

to be tasted and
returned to, at a moment
when I want flavor.

———

DREAM—MEAT COUNTER AND PILE OF TINY, COLORED, DEAD, ADORABLE ELE-
PHANTS. WITHOUT MAGICAL THINKING I IMAGINE THE WORLD WOULD BE
GRAY, NO COLORS, AIR PUSHED OUT OF IT, LIKE A PILE OF DEAD LITTLE ELE-
PHANTS—THE HORROR WAS IN HOW CUTE THEY STILL WERE—ASSOCIATION IS
ALSO TO WOODY GUTHRIE SONG ABOUT THE CHILDREN OF STRIKING MINERS
SMOTHERED IN A CRUSH AND TAKEN BACK UNDER THE CHRISTMAS TREE BY
PARENTS—

———

At first I thought I'd know when therapy was successful because I'd
stop feeling the want of being dead.

But, I finally say to Shannon, "This is such a deep, old fact about
me that it could be a *terrible* index of what might change. If I waited
for that . . . !"

I'm wondering now what else might be different and better—
even for someone who remains convinced, with the ancients, that it
would be best not to be born.

Yes, Shannon says. He too has assumed this is a likely scenario:
many other things changing but the one thing not changing. Also, he
says, if such a thing did change it would probably do so imperceptibly
slowly.

Then he produces an apparent non sequitur. A story about a patient of his long ago, someone with "not exactly multiple personalities,

but I would say that
the parts of her were only
barely holding hands,"

who after many years—in fact long after the end of therapy—woke up one morning and found she no longer had multiples. Just that suddenly.

Looking back, I think he's produced this story "just in case." Just in case, that is, what my announcement really meant was something different, something like "I think I'm ready to relinquish this stubborn symptom, but I'm scared about what will be left of *me*."

I love his floating the story so coolly *as* a non sequitur—a story about the non-necessity, in therapy, of what "follows." It gives me a clue. I want to be open to the chance that what any clamorous pain

> wants to tell me, is
> that it is ready at last
> to bid me goodbye.

After this, in fact, I get very charmed and relaxed by everything that looks like non-necessity. I've started noticing how lots of Shannon's best comments—the ones that change the aspect of things for me— amount to nothing more profound than "It ain't necessarily so."

Nowadays, when students ask me, about one thing or another, "But wouldn't that clearly imply—?" or "Doesn't that have to involve—?" it feels Shannonlike when I can respond,

> that may not be a
> theoretical question.
> Just empirical.

SHIFT! LOOKING THROUGH THE NEW PHONE BOOK, E FINDS OUT THAT MY WIFE IS IN THE SAME PRACTICE WITH ME. SHE IS QUITE ANGRY AND SAD. ABOUT THE ANGER, SHE IS GLAD THAT SHE IS FEELING IT BECAUSE IN OTHER

RELATIONSHIPS WHEN THERE COMES A RIVAL, SHE IS GOOD AT REORIENTING
HERSELF TO RELATING TO A COUPLE, MAKES FRIENDS WITH THE RIVAL, SELDOM
LETS HERSELF EXPERIENCE HER ANGER AT THE LOSS, AND NEVER LETS HERSELF
EXPRESS IT. THE SADNESS (AND THE ANGER) SEEM TO BE ABOUT SEVERAL
THINGS. ONE IS THAT SHE EXPERIENCES A LOSS IN THE NATURE OF THE SPACE
OF THE THERAPY (THE BUILDING), WHICH NOW FEELS LIKE DULL CONJUGAL
SPACE RATHER THAN OUR ADVENTUROUS SPACE. THE NEW INFORMATION
BRINGS HER FACE TO FACE WITH THE REALITY THAT THERE IS SOMEONE ELSE
IN MY LIFE. SHE IDENTIFIES THIS AS AN OEDIPAL SITUATION, BUT MORE
WHERE SHE HAD TO REMEMBER THAT HER MOTHER HAD A HUSBAND THAN
VICE-VERSA. THE OTHER STRUCTURE OF THIS COMES MORE RECENTLY FROM K.C.
AND HER AFFAIR WITH HIM. IN THIS SHE REALIZED THAT SOMEHOW SHE HER-
SELF GAINED AND GREW A LOT IN THE EXPERIENCE, FINDING IT UNIQUE, BUT
THAT FOR HIM IT WAS MOSTLY ANOTHER IN A LINE OF AFFAIRS, SOMETHING OF
AN INTERCHANGEABLE PART, AND THAT WHAT SHE BROUGHT TO THE RELA-
TIONSHIP WITH HIM HE SIMPLY TOOK BACK TO THE MARRIAGE AND USED IT TO
MAKE THE MARRIAGE WORK BETTER FOR HIM. DESPITE THINKING SHE FINALLY
GOT MORE THAN HE FROM THEIR AFFAIR, SHE FEELS HUMILIATED AND DIMIN-
ISHED IN THIS SCENARIO. I TELL HER A LITTLE OF THE FACTUAL INFORMATION
ABOUT MY WIFE'S BEING IN THE PRACTICE. E ALSO SEES IT AS NARROW AND
UNIMAGINATIVE OF ME TO SO ARRANGE MY LIFE, AND TO THE EXTENT SHE
NEEDS ME TO BE "SMARTER," LESS CONVENTIONAL, AND ALSO WISHES FOR ME
TO BE SO, THE FACT THAT I WOULD DO THIS IN MY LIFE IS DISAPPOINTING.

"You know, I'm remembering," I tell Shannon, "a particular point in
my learning about triangular desire, something that came to me in my
late twenties, after a few years with K.C. A notion I thought of as 'post-
Proustian love.'

"Yeah, it comes back. That whereas my earlier ways of identifying
with adulterous romance—like reading *The Once and Future King*, or
seeing *Jules and Jim*—always involved a kind of narrow sexual trian-
gle, or at least a

circuit small enough
that its allure was, you would
eventually

get back all of the
erotic energy you'd
sent around it (so

that the point of this
fantasy was *nothing is*
ever really lost)—

in post-Proustian
love, on the other hand, the
circuit could be big.

Imagine it big
enough that you could never
even *know* whether

the system was closed,
finally, or open. So
the point could only

lie in valuing
all the transformations and
transitivities

in all directions
for their difference, trans-i-ness,
and their skilled nature.

"Not their closure—so that K.C. might get all this care and irony from
his wife—spend it on worry, guilt, and sex with me and whoever
else—receive devotion and rage back from me—but also permit me to

send off, in some other direction, a ratcheted-up level of writing and analysis that might be energizing in some other way to friends or readers or to Hal, who would return nurturance to me and, who knows, frustration and pleasure to someone he might be intimate with, who . . . and so forth and so on."

For some reason, picturing this new kind of circuitry was a vital *self-protective* step for me; somehow it changed what was at stake in the "between"-ness of adultery. Also it made adultery feel less deadeningly heterosexual, moving it toward the (for me) vastly more spacious and inviting field of queerness.

The space of Shannon is both myself and not.

> The place where talking
> to someone else is also
> talking to myself.

I've never experienced this interlocution before.

AN AWKWARD SESSION AS SHE DOES NOT WANT TO SAY GOODBYE FOR THE WEEK PLUS, AND I AM CONCERNED ABOUT HER BEING OK ESPECIALLY WITH THE GO- ING TO CONFERENCE. I REMEMBER THE COUPLE OF TIMES SHE WAS ATTACKED IN CONFERENCES. IN ANY CASE WE MANAGE TO PART, WITH VISITS ON RETURN- ING CLEARLY SCHEDULED.

The hour seems quiet and it occurs to me to ask, as I haven't before, whether Shannon has any idea how obsessively I document our meet- ings. (Not really.) And, by implication, whether he thinks it is a bad idea. (No!)

He volunteers that I seem like someone for whom words have a big ontological importance—like things don't quite exist till I've said them. "Or," I say, "maybe it's more about loss—things *exist* without words, but without words I've no safeguard against losing them the next minute."

It's a pleasure and satisfaction to me to keep a record—as a way of keeping hold of what happens and steeping myself in it.

Shannon says, he also keeps seeing (in his phrase) "my four-year-old girl" (it takes me a second to realize he's talking about something from his repertoire of images of me, not one of his own kids) "my four-year-old girl standing stubbornly in the middle of a room, saying something that's encountered some unexpected opposition, and feeling suddenly how fortifying it would be to have an authoritative record to appeal to, of exactly what had gone before—"

"Yes," I agree with high recognition, "all those topics I'd venture on stoutly, assuming I knew what I was talking about, and only suddenly retrospectively conscious that I absolutely didn't——"

Though, I also say, I don't seem to use this record of our hours so much that way.

One thing it does do is let me indulge that desire, identified by Proust, to *show oneself to be loved*. (A shy glance at Shannon. Yes! He is nodding. As if he agrees that an account of our interactions will *show me to be loved*.)

A bit later, but maybe through the four-year-old, I'm suddenly in mind of the many childhood moments when, for one reason or another, I vowed to myself to remember something or willed to remember it. Specifically: to remember it into adulthood. Whether to bear witness to the pains of childhood, or to make myself behave differently toward kids when I was a grownup, or just—to remember.

In particular I'm now remembering: one patch of dirt in my elementary school yard that (wandering around the periphery one recess, of course instead of playing ball with my agemates) I stood staring at and intensely willing myself, yes, *this* I will remember, *this* I will project forward into the future so that it's there as much as it is here, just *this*, not because it's exceptional but because it's ordinary, it's nothing, it's dirt; I will remember it.

Perspective which keeps opening for me: the distance from age-mates turning into the creation of an inner space (and wasn't it exactly to that inner space that the attention of the future—the future me—was being trained? Like, "This may look like just another little kid, looking back—you may wonder if she has an inner life at all!—but, here's proof: her inner life was powerful enough to conjure *you* up, long before you existed, and install an entirely arbitrary [and hence how signifying!] imprint in your memory)"—an inner space that also, though, *was* the space of the gesture toward the future.

Then suddenly I'm crying. To Shannon's mildly interrogative face: "I guess I'm responding to the distance between recounting it to you, this story, in this context of being loved and listened to—the distance between this and the form of

> memory that girl
> is practicing. Where no such
> conditions obtain."

———————

When I'm away from Shannon, I try to summon it up—the voice that speaks in a quiet double way, the being alone but not alone.

> It is my own soft
> voice. But once I can hear it—
> I'm back with Shannon.

———————

RETURNS WITH A COLD AND "OFF CENTER." SHE RECEIVED ADULATION AT THE CONFERENCE WITH A NUMBER OF PEOPLE TELLING HER WHAT A DIFFERENCE HER WRITING HAS MADE IN THEIR LIVES, ONE YOUNGER GUY SAYING THAT IN-TERVIEWING HER WAS HIGH POINT IN HIS LIFE. SHE IS PLEASED BUT AS USUAL DOESN'T KNOW WHAT TO DO WITH THE PRAISE. IT SEEMS TO MAKE HER ILL AT EASE.

PHYSICALLY A LITTLE BETTER. HAS FOUND HERSELF UNABLE TO DO MUCH PRO-
DUCTIVE WORK SINCE VACATION AND IN REALITY HAS AN IMMENSE AMOUNT OF
WORK AND TRAVEL TO DO IN THE NEXT MONTH OR SO. HEAD COLD COMBINES
WITH THE SENSE OF A WAVE BREAKING OVER HER TO MAKE HER FEEL UNABLE
TO BREATHE.

VERY INTERESTING SESSION. E TALKS SOME ABOUT HER FRIEND GARY (A BLACK
WRITER, EX-STUDENT OF HERS) AND ALSO ABOUT JAMES BALDWIN NOVEL SHE IS
READING. SHE DESCRIBES THE BOOK WHICH CONTAINS THEMES OF PERSONAL
ALIENATION, THE ATTEMPT TO MAINTAIN LOVE AND FAMILY GIVEN THAT AND
THE STRESSES OF OPPRESSION AND RACISM. BESIDES THE TIE-INS TO HER FAM-
ILY, E ALSO TALKS ABOUT HER EMOTIONAL TIES TO BLACK FRIENDS, CULTURE
AND POLITICS. AS I ASK QUESTIONS SHE TALKS ABOUT HAVING COME TO APPRE-
CIATE THE REALITIES OF OPPRESSION, POWER, RACISM, POLITICS, ETC., LATE IN
LIFE (MIDCOLLEGE), AND HER EMOTIONAL SENSE THAT THE PROBLEMS ARE UN-
SOLVABLE FINALLY AND THAT SHE IS AS MUCH PART OF THE PROBLEM AS PART
OF THE SOLUTION, DESPITE HER BEST EFFORTS TO MAKE SOME DIFFERENCE IN
THEM. SHE REALIZES THAT THE KNOWLEDGE OF SYSTEMIC SOCIAL FORCES CAME
LATER BUT THAT THE SENSE OF FATALITY AND THE SENSE OF ACUTE, FEARED
PERSONAL RESPONSIBILITY HAVE EARLIER ROOTS. SHE ALLUDES TO HER SENSE
IN HER FAMILY THAT SHE WAS RESPONSIBLE FOR ITS ??? (SMOOTH FUNCTION-
ING? STABILITY ? HAPPINESS?) BUT ALSO THE CAUSE OF OR CONTRIBUTOR TO
THE DYSFUNCTION OR UNHAPPINESS OR ???

To Tim again: Am in deepish dumps after a really crummy session of
unsweet Shannon unthought. Trying to follow back the thread of
pink-diaper baby EKS and the political performativities of the fifties (I
recounted that a cousin of mine was one of the Unfriendly 10, consequently blacklisted, etc. — and thus that performative silence, Not
Testifying, the potent reticence, *il gran rifiuto*, was part of an obscured

family legend, if not ethic). From there, via Gary, to the subject of race in general, at least the black/white version that we easterners recognize as the subject of race—and all the ways I feel like my upbringing twisted me into a small, tight, raw pretzel around this topic: my family's antiracism, my family's racism, the yawningly abysmal gap of inarticulation between them.

Now for me, this is a wrackingly depressive topic—I mean I don't get anywhere new with it, there's a load of habituated pain, there's a vindictively strong ethical line that never seems to *work*, I feel both wretchedly self-righteous and also a hundred percent in the wrong all the time. And I guess I was listening to Shannon kind of cross-eyed too, because on the one hand I've always seen him as someone who might be of distantly African descent himself, thus maybe observing from a complicated place in terms of his own racial identifications . . . and on the other hand the language he kept coming up with was so bland, complacent, ignorant and uncaring, so sheerly unthoughtful, that it was as if he couldn't see the point of the topic at all.

(Specifically—can I make myself tell you this?—the brilliant reflections he was producing included things like, that the problem he has thinking about race is that he can't keep track of what people want to call themselves . . . They aren't black anymore, are they? . . . Certainly not Negro . . . African-Americans? People of color? Who can keep up with these things? Along those illuminating lines! Also, when I sounded savage about my parents' double-binding racial attitudes he asked innocently whether that wasn't just something like an intermediate phase of evolution, like animals with wings and scales . . . and that whites of, say, our generation would just kind of *naturally* be more evolved in our attitudes about race.

I mean it wasn't *so* bad, not evil, but it was . . . dumb! Indifferent!)

After a while I asked in dismay, "It does make sense for me to talk about these things, doesn't it?"

And he said, numbly or apathetically, "I don't know, it might." About to die from the tedium.

So I am feeling both as though I'm completely inadequate as a patient and also totally let down by him.

And everything just seems so dead.

I wouldn't have thought, even a few hours ago, that things could feel this way so suddenly.

He could tell it was a bad place to leave me in ("Here we are at one of those awful stopping places").

But, oh, the little
histrionics of the dropped
patient at hour's end . . .

———

And later to Tim: Still been trying to process the stuff with Shannon. But trying not to try too hard—I sort of wasn't up for the version where I get it all figured out and report to him why he's not really such an asshole after all and why it's all really Interesting.

(Still, it *is* interesting, isn't it?—that the absolute laying low of my opinion of him, and of myself, were so entirely tied up in each other, and so sudden?)

———

And this time, an hour with Shannon gets me back on the rails.

I must admit there's some fun in being able to say all my meanest things to him, only slightly cloaked in the sad severity of free indirect discourse. Like, "When I walked out of here Monday, I don't know which was lower, my opinion of you or of myself. I was feeling that everything you said was a tissue of evasive clichés. What an idiot! I was thinking," and on and on. I have the sense that he sort of relishes my relish, actually. (I don't know if it's better or worse that a lot of it gets cast in the third person: "I thought, Shannon's never done anything in his life that I would count as *thinking*!")

But the sense that he'll be able to weather this storm of devaluation—that stays rock solid. And I do feel I've managed to hold on to a striking finding: though I was savaging him and myself for different reasons—his unthoughtfulness, my shaming inability to capture his interest—in fact the collapse within me of his stock and my stock was not only simultaneous but, it seems clearly, the same thing.

And Shannon rewards me, not just by not withering up in the face of my scorn, not just either by not withering me (which he could easily do, though not I think with scorn . . . just by seeming bored, say), but by asking me this. ("I know this is a funny question.")

"The way your evaluation of yourself and of me were all knotted together," he says, "makes it sound as if this all comes from some situation you felt you couldn't get out of. Yeah? So let me ask you this, if it makes any sense: imagine if you hadn't been able to walk out of here after an hour on Monday. Imagine that we'd just kept sitting here doing what we were doing all afternoon."

"Oh, I think we could have really gotten somewhere!" I offer brightly.

"No," he says, "but if we weren't able to stop doing whatever it was that was so awful. If we'd just kept doing it and doing it—

"What would it have felt like to you to have to keep talking to somebody that dumb? I mean, would it have felt more like talking to somebody angry? Or somebody depressed? Or somebody dead? Or what?"

> When someone gets blank
> in that particular way,
> so tied to l'idée
>
> reçue, it's true—it
> does feel like assault. And, yes
> also it's like a
>
> kind of depressive
> stonewalling. And in the way
> that, dealing with the
>
> dead, you always want
> to tell them to just come off
> it—resume being

recognizable
to you, and recognizing
you—that being dumb

and dead can both seem
like cheap tricks for refusing
recognition—yes,

it does seem a braid of the three; a familiar one, banefully.

———————

How they're intertwined—
his permanence in me—my
permanence in him—

How, when I suppose
him to be forgetting or
dropping me—somehow—

from his mind—I lose
the Daedalian thread of
Shannon in *my* mind—

———————

Back from the hour, I find a present from my folks: the catalogue of
an Egon Schiele show at the National Gallery, inscribed

"to our favorite
poet and dear daughter, Eve."
It moves me so much—

Invoking the identity "poet" for me is one of the very oldest of ges-
tures among my family. The "dear daughter, Eve" part of it speaks

somehow, eloquently for me, of the more recent past: the sense for the last some number of years that my folks felt maybe even an unexpected increase in the way of love (this I think largely the result of Nina's brutalizing silent treatment of them for so many years—it made them very tender toward me and David). Yet I note too the humble parental care to distinguish that though I'm their "favorite poet," even now they would never choose a "favorite daughter"—only distinguish a "dear" one. I am saying "they" here, but of course this inscription is my mother's.

———————

It's a spring day, mild and rainy, when I'm walking on campus, an inward smile on my inward face, glad I'll be seeing Shannon soon. Besides the pleasure of the prospect, there's a little anxiety about whether I'll be able to get centered and at home with him promptly; whether whatever it is I have in mind to mention will open onto something interesting to us both or not.

The strange form of address is taking shape in my head again, the unmistakable one that's somewhere between talking to myself and talking to another person.

But invoking Shannon's wide sheltered room in this wet, calm outdoor space is centering me already—centers me, it seems, with a quiet inside voice that is noting,

> I can tune my mind today
> to the story I think I want to tell you;
> I can tune my eyes
> already to your face, listening.

As indeed, I can.

As I walk, I guess my little smile is enfolding a new thought: when I get inside maybe I'll put these words on a scrap of paper and see whether they look (as they sort of sound to me) like the possible start of a poem.

Years since I've tasted this particular mild, speculative smile, isn't it?

———————

"PARANOID" SCENE OF MY WIFE, SEVERE, COMING INTO THE WAITING ROOM, LOOKING TO E REPROACHFUL. E FEELS ALREADY IN THE WRONG. ONE STRANGE PART IS THAT SHE THINKS OF THE DYNAMIC WITH HER MOTHER AS BEING ABOUT THE TWO OF THEM, NOT TRIANGULAR. I ASK WHO I AM IN THIS. E DOES NOT KNOW. SAYS IF THERE WAS SUCH A THING AS A GOOD CARETAKING MOTHER IT WAS HER MOTHERING HER MOTHER PIECED TOGETHER WITH PIECES OF THE CARETAKING OF OTHERS. I ASK WHERE THE REPROACH COMES IN. E INITIALLY SAYS IT IS THE REPROACH OF MY WIFE, KNOWING HOW MUCH OF ME AND MY TIME AND ATTENTION E WANTS; THAT IT IS A ZERO-SUM GAME WHERE ANYTHING SHE GETS IS TAKEN FROM MY WIFE. THEN SHE SAYS IT IS MORE HER OWN REPROACH AND ANGER AT HER MOTHER— "WHERE WERE YOU?!?"

———————

ISSUE WITH MY WIFE RAISES FOR HER THE ISSUE OF POSSIBLE CHANGES IN HER RELATIONSHIPS WITH WOMEN, WHICH SHE SEES AS THE BIGGEST UNADDRESSED ISSUE OF THERAPY. SAYS THAT UP TO A CERTAIN POINT SHE HAS A LOT OF WARMTH AND TRUST WITH WOMEN AS LONG AS SHE CAN STAY IN AN ADULT POSITION, BE SELF-POSSESSED, THE WOMAN NOT BE CRITICAL OR REPROACHING, AND AS LONG AS THE EROTIC POTENTIAL STAYS DIFFUSE. I COMMENT ON THE PRECARIOUSNESS OF THIS POSITION. E SAYS IT IS PRECARIOUS BECAUSE OF THE POSSIBILITY OF BETRAYAL—BETRAYING OR BEING BETRAYED. THIS SEEMS TO BE THE ISSUE OF REAL OR NONREAL ATTENTION, SPONTANEITY OR LACK OF. SHE TALKED ABOUT ITS BEING IMPORTANT TO BE LOYAL TO YOUR OWN GENDER. REALIZES THAT SHE FEELS TO BE FEMALE IS A SOLID GENDER POSITION, THAT ONE IS FEMALE, THE ONLY QUESTIONS BEING IF YOU ARE A FAILURE IN LIVING UP TO SOME STANDARD OF FEMALENESS OR FEMININITY. IN CONTRAST, TO BE MALE IS LESS SOLID; MORE POSSIBLE TO BE "NOT A MAN." SHE REALIZES THAT THIS DOES NOT EXPLAIN WHY WOMEN "SO SHED MY ATTENTION, TRUST AND LOVE." I AM WONDERING IF WE SHOULD LOOK AT THIS IN TERMS OF HER FEARING GET-

TING PULLED INTO SOME AVERSIVE ROLE WITH WOMEN, OR WHETHER IN A RE-
LATIONSHIP WITH A WOMAN SHE IS AFRAID OF ENCOUNTERING SOME AVOIDED
PART OF HERSELF. E SAYS THAT IN RELATIONSHIP WITH WOMEN SHE FEELS SHE
DISSOLVES, STOPS BEING HERSELF (IS SHE STILL EVEN A WOMAN?), IS AFRAID
OF NOT BEING, OF NOT HAVING A SELF, OF BEING INADEQUATE, NEGLIGIBLE.
WITH "PEOPLE WHO ARE NOT WOMEN" SHE FEELS SPECIAL, VERY POWERFUL AND
PLENTIFUL. WITH WOMEN SHE FEELS NO SPECIAL POWER AND LOTS OF AT SEA IN
EMOTIONAL STUFF. // SOMEWHERE IN HERE WE ALSO TOUCH ON E'S CONSUM-
MATE TENDENCY—HAVING LEARNED/REALIZED/FELT THAT SHE WOULD LOSE IF
SHE COMPETED ON SOMEONE ELSE'S TURF (GIVING UP THE OEDIPAL STRUGGLE
IN HOPELESSNESS) SHE LEARNS TO FIND A THIRD ALTERNATIVE TO COMPETING
OR GIVING UP—TO CREATE HER OWN TURF, A GROUND THAT IS JUST HERS, BUT
THEN SHE CAN MAKE PROFFER OF IT TO OTHERS.

REALIZATION: IT'S NOT ME WHO'S PARANOID, IT'S MY MOTHER, ABOUT ME
(WARY, FEARFUL OF BEING DEPLETED, FEARFUL OF REPROACH). WHEN E EXPE-
RIENCES PARANOIA IT FEELS ALIEN RATHER THAN SYNTONIC.—SHE IS INTER-
ESTED IN THE BOLLAS CONCEPT OF "GENERA," SOMETHING YOU FIGURE OUT
EARLY THAT BECOMES THE NODE OF LATER CREATIVE SKILLS. LIKE HER INSIS-
TENCE ON BOTH/AND THINKING RATHER THAN EITHER/OR. E ASSOCIATES THIS
WITH "TAURUS" REFUSAL TO RELINQUISH OBJECTS. HER MOTHER APPEARS TO
DO THE BOTH/AND, BUT, RATHER THAN SYNTHESIZING OR GETTING TO A POSSI-
BLE NEW PLACE, MORE OFTEN SETTLES ON A PARALYZING PARADOX OR UNRE-
SOLVABLE AMBIGUITY THAT DOESN'T MOVE FURTHER. MOM SEEMS TO LOVE
PARADOX, E DOES NOT AT ALL. E'S INSISTENCE ON EMERGING INTO SOME
OTHER KIND OF RESOLUTION ABUTS HER MAGICAL THINKING AT THIS POINT.

E-mailing Tim: "Quite a lot of water under the bridge, and welling up
over it, since I broke off to answer the phone a couple of hours ago. It
was my folks. Had just heard from Stanley, my sister Nina's husband,
by phone. (This is my sister—I've told you about her, I know—who's

been incommunicado from any of us for a couple of decades. And we don't really know why. In spite of that—or, obviously, because—a huge, silent presence to us all.)

"Now today happens to be Nina's birthday, so I'm certain she was already on my parents' minds. And Stanley tells them: (1) Nina now wants to be back in contact with them. (But it was he, not she, who was calling. And where was she? "Not here right now.") And, (2) Stan himself is very ill. It sounds as though a melanoma he had many years ago has metastasized to his lymph system, or some system anyhow; they didn't get a clear account, but at any rate it is metastatic, hence presumably incurable.

"Stan is—what—forty-six or forty-seven?

"His doctor is trying to get him into a clinical trial at NIH, only a few blocks from my parents' house in Bethesda. And he'll know in a few days. Will call back then.

"We call this: Mixed Feelings."

"I just feel exhausted," I'm telling Shannon. "I feel like a pinball in the middle of a long game. No more happened today; but I feel I haven't begun to process what's happening with Nina and Stan. And I still basically don't know what's going on."

Shannon asks me if there's anything I'd like him to do.

"Could you please make things stop happening," I suggest wanly— he doesn't volunteer to do so—"and if you could sort of glue me to the ground so I don't just get buffeted away?"

"That would be the worst thing I could do," he says. "With these waves coming at you, you need

to be able to
keep bobbing around on the
surface like a cork.

If I glue you to the ground, you'll drown in a minute."

ANOTHER MURDER DREAM—HAD KILLED SOMEONE—HAD TO GIVE A PAPER
ON THE SUBJECT—NO ONE SUSPECTED HER—Q OF HOW MUCH SHOULD SHE
SAY—ENDED UP SAYING NOTHING ABOUT IT IN THE PAPER. LEGALISTIC TONE /
SCARY / INDICTABLE. LETTING SOMEONE/SOMETHING DIE DREAMS AND KILLING
SOMEONE DREAMS FEEL THE SAME—AGENCY IS UNCLEAR—RESPONSIBILITY IS
ON HER ALWAYS. //

Hard to believe there's more bad news right away. This doesn't even count as unexpected: getting back from somebody's dinner party, there's a message from Gary saying he's in the hospital in Berkeley—he's been in there for a week—with, he says, CMV in the gut.

I can't remember much about CMV. I know it's what makes people with AIDS go blind. I don't remember hearing of it in the intestines.

Gary says, in the message, that they think it's probably what was causing that terrible cough. And that they've "isolated" it, presumably meaning there is something they can at least try to do.

He sounds very sick, still hacking, very weak. Says it's been grueling.

I can't tell what he thinks is happening. He talks about finding a new apartment "after he gets out of the hospital." But he also says he has the story he promised to send me, and a letter to me he still wants to "revise," at the hospital with him, and he "promises not to die before he sends them."

And says he loves me and he wishes things had been different so there would have been more chance to show it.

(Though he does show it.)

I feel caught in a high wind with this one.

Want to go straight
to him. And want to run to
the opposite ends

of the earth rather
than feel even closer to him
before I lose him.

———

"I had a good talk with my folks this afternoon. I called them, just to see how they were processing it all. They seemed startled but glad.

"I said to them, 'It's really disorienting to feel so sad, so excited, so wary, all at the same time.' My father said, 'Yes, and we're feeling all three of those things.'

"Which was a relief. I'd wanted to know, to satisfy myself, that wary *is* one of the things they've been feeling."

Folly! How could I
think they needed to be taught
wariness—by me?

"Also for them to know I'm with them in this whole range of feelings."

Yet it seems so much more real and terrifying, the danger of someone I don't know well—related by no blood and not much of a past—but who loves me and lets me be in relation to him.

"The opposite of my sister; I could probably—with some work—make a list of every time and place I've ever been with Gary. Certainly I could give a summary of the, say, four conversations that have been turning points in our relationship.

"Yet the yearning and fear around him are accessible to me, directly, *as* emotions, about a hundred times more clearly and less baffledly than anything, anything I've felt about Nina in the past two decades. Including the past thirty-six hours."

Shannon wonders, with some tenderness: "You're surprised?"

———

Strange to be plunged again into that set of feelings—

> not quite terror—but
> fright, intense fright; for someone
> else, at a distance.

"I found myself dizzy with it, not paralyzed but very constrained—yes, like being physically constrained—talking with Gary at the hospital this afternoon."

There, it was morning.

He sounding terribly weak.

DREAM WHICH SHE SEES AS UNUSUAL IN THAT IT HAS ANXIETY BUT NO PEOPLE. SHE IS IN THE MIDDLE OF THE OCEAN, NO COAST IN SIGHT, BUT THE WATER IS SHALLOW ENOUGH SHE CAN TOUCH BOTTOM, BUT HER HEAD IS AT WAVE LEVEL. WAVES ARE COMING FROM ALL DIRECTIONS, MOVING HER GENTLY, SOMETIMES BREAKING BEFORE THEY REACH HER, SOMETIMES AFTER. EXTREME ANXIETY IS THE SENSE THAT INEVITABLY A WAVE WILL BREAK RIGHT WHERE SHE IS, UPSETTING HER, PUSHING HER DOWN, TUMBLING HER IN THE SAND AND SHELL PIECES, SHE WOULD GET SMASHED UP. THE SENSATIONS IN THE DREAM ARE VERY PHYSICAL.

Shannon is being silly today. Most of the other shrinks are out of town on holiday, and we joke about running around and taking over other people's offices—my suggestion.

He's glad to hear some better news of Gary, but what he really wants is the dope on my sister. I tell him my folks called Stan yesterday and said they are going away for three weeks on Sunday, so . . .

"So they left him your phone number!?"

"You got it in one."

Big, big wheezy laugh from Shannon.

Then: "What a wicked laugh! Why did I make such a wicked laugh?"

Then: "I guess I *like* this stuff with your sister. It makes . . . you know . . . it makes . . ."

"The kettle simmer?"

"Yeah! The kettle simmer!

"But also, there's a part of me that can't help imagining everything turning out happily. I know that isn't the likeliest thing in the world, but I can't help imagining it: you, your sister, your parents, all restored to one another . . ."

And more along these lines. Which I, truthfully, am finding hard to take.

It does have the merit of shaking me to my senses a little bit, sharpening my own definition:

"You know," I finally say, "I need to tell you, restoring an intact family of origin is not at the top of my list of priorities. In fact, I'd say it's probably on the list of things I don't want to happen."

"Really? I can see why it might not be a priority, but why would you not want it to happen?"

"Well, I can see that maybe I need to piece together a history. But I don't see why I need an intact family now, in the present. And everything in my whole life, since I've had any say about it, has been about a completely different principle of affiliation.

"Like, people who come or stay together because they love each other—can give each other pleasure—have real needs from each other. Not structured around blood and law.

"I hate the idea

    that you're born sewn up
    in a burlap bag with a
    few other creatures,

    and you have to claw
    and fight inside that burlap
    bag for your whole life.

Say, you argue over Grandma's silver after the funeral and don't speak to each other for the next twenty years. And at the end of twenty years, the main thing you're doing with your life is still—not speaking to each other."

Talk about visiting Atlanta sets the stage for a nicely phatic moment.

As we're rising to go, Shannon says to me, or starts to say, "I know you're good, but . . ."

"Oh," I respond, "I'm very, very *good.*"

(I think when he started the sentence, "good" meant something like "effective," in the way a shrink might be effective, on a scene such as the one in Atlanta. My own "good" was more like, I'm a very, very Good Child.)

". . . but not *that* good!" he
concludes. Just as ". . . but there are
limits!" I conclude

—amid hilarity.

On the phone Nina says, I guess it was kind of

retarded to think
Mommy could just come and make
everything all right.

I can't begin to tally the heartbreaking things about this sentence.

7

GENERALLY GOOD WEEKEND W/ NINA ALTHOUGH E FELT "HAUNTED" IN A WAY
SHE CANNOT OTHERWISE DESCRIBE—THE SENSE OF BEING UNABLE TO TELL SIS
AND HAL APART AT SOME STRANGE LEVEL. SIS TALKED SOME @ CHILDHOOD—
HER FEELING THAT SHE WAS RESTRICTED/PRESSED BY PARENTS' RULES, HER
SENSE THAT MOTHER WAS UNCOMFORTING. NOTED THAT FATHER WAS THE
SPANKER WHEN NECESSARY BUT NOT VERY OFTEN. OF MORE INTEREST TO E
WERE SIS'S OBSERVATIONS ON HER DAUGHTER WHOM SHE IDENTIFIES AS
GIFTED. THIS SEEMS TO HAVE ALLOWED SIS TO SEE E IN MORE PERSPECTIVE. AT
END OF HOUR RECOUNTS INCIDENT IN CAR W/ HAL SAYING TO BROTHER-IN-
LAW THAT IF HE CAN CONTINUE TO LIVE FOR A WHILE MEDICAL SCIENCE IS
COMING UP W/ THERAPIES FOR CANCER EVERY DAY. E HEARS THIS AS AIMED AT
HER AND IS ANGRY AS SHE DOES NOT WANT TO LIVE TO OLD AGE BUT DIE
SOONER; ESPECIALLY MUST DIE BEFORE HAL.

There's a funny instant when I'm facing my sister for the first time—

    her so very thin,
    me so very fat—and I
    think we both grasp at

once that through eighteen
years' separation, each girl
must have looked in the

mirror every
morning to see, fearfully,
the other's body.

––––––––––

RE NINA'S DAUGHTER AND "GIFTED CHILDREN," E HAS BEEN THINKING ABOUT
THE TENSION BETWEEN PATIENCE AND IMPATIENCE GIVEN BEING GIFTED—
HOW SHE IS OFTEN IMPATIENT AND SIMPLY HAS LEARNED TO SUPPRESS
HERSELF/ HER VITALITY/ HER IDEAS/ HER IMPATIENCE—AND HOW "VIOLENT"
THIS IS. "*ALL* THAT TIME WAITING FOR OTHER PEOPLE TO FINISH SENTENCES
WHEN YOU ALREADY KNOW WHAT THEY'LL SAY!" HER ATTITUDES OF SECRET CON-
TEMPT ARE TIED UP IN THIS. AS SHE TALKS ABOUT THIS HER IMAGE IS OF A CAT
PLAYING W/ A DEAD MOUSE TO MAKE IT SEEM ALIVE. I LAUGH AND SHE BECOMES
ANXIOUS—PERHAPS BECAUSE SHE HAS EXPRESSED SOME OF THE CONTEMPT
&/OR BECAUSE I'VE SEEN IT. WE TALK MORE AND SHE IS MORE ANXIOUS. I SAY I
FEEL THE CONTEMPT WAS PROBABLY NOT ORIGINALLY PART OF THE FEELING OF
BEING GIFTED OR IMPATIENT. SHE CHANGES TOPIC TO ASK @ MY REACTION TO
THE END OF LAST SESSION (NEED TO DIE BEFORE HAL). I TELL HER MY VARIOUS
ASSOCIATIONS—SHE WAS INTERESTED BECAUSE SHE HAS NOT SAID THIS BEFORE
SO CLEARLY AND WONDERED HOW IT SOUNDED TO ME.

––––––––––

Isn't hope the most bewildering of emotions?

Painful as it is, I can't help feeling it about Nina, about my parents.
But how fraying to experience that hope at the same time as the feelings for Gary,

which seem to offer
joys of a deepening and
deepening friendship

on only this one,
simple, wee condition: that
I may never hope.

———————

SAT. NIGHT FEELING HAL WAS MY SISTER CLIMBED INTO MY BED AT NIGHT—
SPOOKY—AM I A CHILD OR AN ADULT?—AM I A SEPARATE BEING?—LIKE I
DON'T EXIST IN THE SPACE BETWEEN MY MOTHER AND NINA—I FEEL LIKE I'M
NOT THERE.

———————

E ASSOCIATES NINA WITH DISGUST, WITH HAVING BEEN UNABLE TO INDIVIDU-
ATE AND HENCE HAVING SWALLOWED "SOMETHING BAD" (HER MOTHER), WITH
HER FACE EXPRESSING DISGUST OFTEN. SHE ALSO REMEMBERS FINDING THINGS
ABOUT N AS A TEEN—HAIR IN THE SINK, POWDER ON THE BLOUSE—DISGUST-
ING—THE TRACES OF N. MOTHER'S AFFECT IS DISTASTE RATHER THAN DISGUST
—MOTHER SEEMINGLY EXPERIENCES BODY AS PRISTINE, PREPUBESCENT, BOY-
ISH, DRY.—TALKS ABOUT THE POSITION OF BEING BETWEEN N AND MOTHER AS
ONE SHE SHOULD GET OUT OF, ONE THAT HAS LITTLE IN IT FOR HER.

"It's deeply haunting to me to be with my sister. I really do think it
must be true that a lot of boundaries between me and not-me fall, not
between me and my mother, but me and Nina.

"When I've been with her there's

some clinging presence
around me, or a voice, or
a scent, or feeling

about which I can't tell whether it's mine or another's. Or it's like a big self and a little, supplementary other person; or vice versa. I can't describe it, but it's so real. It's truly the *unheimlich*, I guess.

"Of course it feels ordinary as bread."

—————

THE STORY OF THE BREAKFAST FIGHTS AND HOW TOTALLY E HATES EGGS WHICH MOTHER MADE HER EAT EVERY OTHER DAY. BESIDES WHY MOTHER DID THIS— E JUST GOES ON AND ON ABOUT ALL THE WAYS EGGS ARE DISGUSTING.

—————

NINA AND THEIR MOTHER HATED EGGS TOO!! MOTHER WOULD GET NAUSEATED, RETCHING, GAGGING WHEN FIXING THEM (BUT INSISTED ON FIXING THEM). MOTHER AS HYSTERICAL IN THE SELF PSYCHOLOGY SENSE AND IN THE CLASSIC FREUDIAN SENSE OF BEING OUT OF TOUCH WITH HER BODY WHILE STILL TYING THINGS BACK THROUGH HER BODY TO EXPRESS WHATEVER SHE DID NOT OTH-ERWISE EXPRESS OR DIRECTLY FEEL. BODY—MOTHER COULD TOTALLY SUBLI-MATE HER BODY, TURN IT INTO AIR (ALWAYS DRESSED IN SUMMER CLOTHES) BUT E DIDN'T HAVE THAT KIND OF BODY.

—————

NINA'S FEELINGS OF BEING UNABLE TO DO THINGS RIGHT, AND OF A PECULIAR DISCOMFORT ATTENDANT ON INTERACTIONS WITH HER MOTHER. FOR EXAMPLE, THE CONVERSATIONS ABOUT MOTHER'S FRIENDS, USUALLY CRITICAL, THAT E RE-MEMBERS AS TIMES SHE JOINED WITH HER MOTHER IN PLEASURABLE, EXCITING ADULT-SOUNDING ("PSYCHOANALYZING") TALK, N REMEMBERS AS CONFUSING AND HOSTILE. SHE AND E CONCUR ON THEIR MOTHER'S WONT TO SUDDENLY DISENGAGE AND BE ABSENT OR BE IN AN ENTIRELY DIFFERENT PLACE (LIKE WHAT AM I DOING TALKING TO YOU ABOUT THIS?). N REINFORCES THE IMPOR-TANCE OF SIZE IN THE FAMILY—THAT IT MADE A BIG DIFFERENCE WHEN E BE-CAME BIGGER THAN SHE WAS, A CHANGE SHE REMEMBERS HAPPENING WHEN

SHE WAS ABOUT 6 AND E 3!! SHE ALSO PAINTS E IN CHILDHOOD WITH INTER-
ESTING PHRASES—FROM ANOTHER PLANET, A BABY BUDDHA, SOMEHOW SEEN
TO UNDERSTAND BOTH FACTUAL AND EMOTIONAL THINGS IN AN UNCANNY
AND INTUITIVE WAY THAT ASTOUNDED. SHE FELT A SENSE OF PROTECTIVENESS,
COMPETITIVENESS, MYSTIFICATION, SOME AWE AT E. SHE WONDERS WHAT IT
WAS LIKE FOR HER BEFORE E CAME ALONG.

My dictionary
entries for *distrait*: distraught,
distressed, distracted.

Shannon and I agree: feeling "not together" is part of the bobbing-
like-a-cork strategy. Temporarily disarticulating my different worlds
from each other, my faculties, my past from present from future.

How are you bearing it, he asks me later—the death that's all around
you? Isn't the oppression of it too much for you?

But after a month or two, my image of it is different. Stan is dying.
Nina has reappeared as in a Shakespearean romance. Gary is dying.
But then, my poetry has returned. And returning with it, and with
Shannon's escort, is some of the long-ago life of the girl whose first
passion it was. What it's feeling like to me isn't death, but a great, up-
welling flux of mutability

as if, falling in,
you'd emerge young—old—dead—a
different person—

E IN THE MIDST OF WRITING A PAPER AND CONSEQUENTLY OUT OF TOUCH
WITH HER INTERNAL LIFE. AT MY ASKING, TALKS ABOUT THE PAPER. IT IS FASCI-

NATING TO ME TO GET A LOOK INTO HER FORMULATING THESE IDEAS; THE
IDEAS ARE QUITE INTERESTING; MOSTLY IT IS JUST NICE TO SEE HER SO EN-
GROSSED AND ENJOYING HERSELF IN THIS QUITE SATISFYING WAY.

———

Shannon and I both read James Merrill, and I'm quoting to him from
Ephraim, the small-caps-speaking spirit summoned through a Ouija
board in *Divine Comedies*—

                                   FOR
NOTHING LIVE IS MOTIONLESS HERE OUR STATE IS EXCITING AS
WE MOVE WITH THE CURRENT & EMOTION BECOMES AN ELEMENT
OF ITS OWN FORCE O MY I AM TOO EXCITED. . . .
. . . NOW U UNDERSTAND MY LOVE OF TELLING MY LIFE
FOR IN ALL TRUTH I AM IMAGINING THAT NEXT ONE WHEN WE
CRASH THROUGH IN OUR NUMBERS TRANSFORMING LIFE INTO
WELL EITHER A GREAT GLORY OR GREAT PUDDLE

———

FELT LOW AFTER MON—ASHAMED, ANXIOUS, FEELING THAT SHE WASN'T ABLE
TO MOVE TOWARD BEING MORE IN TOUCH WITH HER OWN INTERNAL LIFE, OR
TOWARD ME, AND THAT THAT KIND OF ABSORPTION IN HER OWN THOUGHTS
AND IDEAS IS WRONG. THE STRANGENESS OF BEING AT THIS POINT IN A WRIT-
ING PROJECT. BELIEVES SHE HAS BEEN DREAMING OF MOTHER AND SISTER—
THAT A BETRAYAL OF HER SISTER IS IN THE VICINITY OF HER ABILITY TO BE
WRITING AT ALL.

———

POSSIBILITY OF SAYING TO PARENTS THAT SHE DOES NOT WANT TO BE A CON-
DUIT FOR INFORMATION BETWEEN THEM AND NINA—THE PROSPECT PROMPTS
A LOT OF AGONIZING AND ANXIOUS FEELING FOR E. WHAT IF SHE DID DO
SOMETHING THAT ALIENATED HER MOTHER??!!

NOTES HOW CURLED UP SHE GOT LAST HOUR—SMALL TARGET, UNDOING EX-
PANSIVENESS, EXHIBITIONISTIC, HIDING, DISTRESS, DISGUST? WANTS PARENTS
TO LIVE FOREVER BUT ALSO FEELS MOTHER'S IMPINGEMENT ON HER. OPPRESSED
BY THE SENSE OF THERE BEING NO PLACE FOR HER BODY IN THAT FAMILY. SENSE
OF BEING IDENTIFIED WITH MOTHER, IDENTIFIED WITH NINA—NEVER IDEN-
TIFIED WITH HERSELF, EVACUATED, NO SENSE OF HOW TO EXIST THERE. "MY
MOTHER IS REALLY SCARED OF ME." FOCUS ON HER BODY—FLOATING APART
TO DIFFUSE A GENITAL BURNING. "JUST WANT MOTHER TO BE BIGGER," BIG
ENOUGH TO HOLD HER, BIG ENOUGH TO FIGHT WITH HER, BUT MOTHER JUST
GETS SMALLER. THE CONSTANT, ACTIVE REASSURING OF HER MOTHER IS TAXING.
RECALLS HOW IN HS WHEN SHE WAS SO VERY DEPRESSED SHE WORKED HARD TO
REASSURE HER PARENTS THAT HER UNHAPPINESS WASN'T ABOUT THEM, THAT
HER ANGER WASN'T ABOUT THEM.

"I have to keep remembering how different your family is from what
I'm used to! I see the traces of it in so many ways. It's not something
I've seen fifteen or sixteen of. When I imagine the Kosofsky world, it's
like some planet that's

> almost exactly
> the same as here except for
> a few little things—

like, the sky's aqua, and the grass is yellow instead of green, and all the
trees have smooth bark."

DREAM—HUGE OCEAN WAVE CRASHES OVER A SHOPPING MALL PARKING
GARAGE. SHE IS SCARED. SHE FEELS SHE HAS BEEN HAVING OTHER ANXIETY
WAVE DREAMS LIKE THIS LATELY. BUT SHE HAS ALSO BEEN HAVING A CONTINU-

ING IF EPISODIC RECONNECTION WITH THE DIFFUSE SENSE OF SEXUALITY. THE
SENSE IS THAT IT IS THERE LIKE HER INNER VOICE IF SHE CAN QUIET THE
NOISE OF DAILY PROJECTS, THOUGHTS, ANXIETIES. BUT STILL SHE HAS FELT
ANXIOUS/ THE SENSE THAT BAD THINGS COULD HAPPEN AT ANY MOMENT, ESPE-
CIALLY IF SHE IS SCATTERED, NOT CENTERED, NOT ON WATCH. (THIS IS OCCA-
SIONED BY OUR HAVING CHANGED THE APPOINTMENT TIME FOR TODAY, HER
HAVING FORGOT AND COME AN HOUR EARLY, BUT MY HAVING THOUGHT SHE
MIGHT DO SO AND COME THEN MYSELF.) SHE TRIES TO ARTICULATE THE ANXI-
ETY. SOME SHE IS TOUCHED BY MY THOUGHTFULNESS AND PULLED INTO THE
THOUGHT THAT OUR MINDS ARE ATTUNED TO THAT EXTENT. BUT SHE ALSO
FEELS THAT HER SCATTEREDNESS IS PULLING ME OFF CENTER. SHE INTERRUPTS
TO REMEMBER THAT HER FRIEND STEPHEN HAS GIVEN HER A PLAY ABOUT
MELANIE KLEIN AND HER RELATIONSHIP WITH HER DAUGHTER AND A
PROSPECTIVE PATIENT. A PART OF THIS IS HOW TRANSPARENTLY INTERPENE-
TRATED THEIR PSYCHES ARE. I ASK IF THAT HAS SOMETHING TO DO WITH THE
ANXIETY.

––––––––

STILL FEELING STRANGE ABOUT LAST TIME——ANXIETY, INCOMPETENCE,
STRANGE TO HER THAT MY ACTIONS, WHICH SHE FOUND TOUCHING, MADE HER
SO ANXIOUS. SHE RECALLS THAT SHE HAS ALWAYS LIKED IT THAT I DO LITTLE
PRAISING OF HER, THAT I FEEL IMPARTIAL. THERE IS SOMETHING VERY CALM-
ING TO HER ABOUT THE SENSE OF HAVING NO EFFECTS. SHE HAS BEEN ABLE TO
FEEL ABOUT ME WHAT BALINT DESCRIBES OF THE THERAPIST——THAT I PROVIDE
SUPPORT LIKE BUOYANCY IN WATER——THERE, UNFAILING, NOT CARING. SHE
REFLECTS THAT MY COMING EARLY WAS NOT IN RESPONSE TO ANY WISH FROM
HER AS SHE HAD NOT REALIZED THAT SHE WAS EARLY——THAT THERE IS SOME-
THING DANGEROUS IN BEING OFFERED SOMETHING GRATUITOUSLY.

––––––––

THINKING ABOUT CONDITIONAL AND UNCONDITIONAL LOVE CONTINUUM.
FROM K.C. IT WAS QUITE CONDITIONAL, FROM HAL ALMOST ENTIRELY UNCONDI-
TIONAL. FROM BENJ, APPARENTLY CONDITIONAL BUT MORE, IT WAS MAN-

GLINGLY ARBITRARY. FROM ME IT IS UNCONDITIONAL BUT ALSO IS NOT QUITE
LOVE. SHE FINDS SOMETHING USEFUL IN LEAVING IT UNDEFINED OR NOT
QUITE DEFINED AS LOVE. THE UNCONDITIONAL WHATEVER FEELS MOST CENTER-
ING TO HER.

———

Learning so well and early to do, emotionally, for myself . . . in a way
it worked splendidly; in a way it really didn't.

Shannon's interrogative glance.

"Well, here I am, aged forty-four, and completely hung up on my
mother!

"Also, think how inefficient it is, this way of keeping one's own self
consolidated and comforted. Which is great for some things. I expect
its wastefulness has a lot to do with how floppy, productive, represen-
tational—for some other people too—that 'self' turns out to be. It has

> a big, loose footprint
> like a messy hurricane—
> it churns up the space—
>
> and maybe it keeps
> things aerated and fertile.
> (Though it's such hard work.)

———

At the end of the hour, though, only a single discovery has stuck in my
mind.

> It's true, isn't it?
> I *am* pathetically in
> love with my mother.

Shannon deprecates
"pathetic." But pathetic's
part of what I *like*—

E TALKED WITH HER PARENTS WHO WILL BE VISITING THE EARLY PART OF NEXT
MONTH AND THEY ARE WILLING TO MEET WITH ME. THIS WILL BE WITHOUT E
AND INDIVIDUALLY WITH EACH PARENT, AT THE REQUEST OF HER MOTHER.
E FORMULATES THE FACT THAT "I HAVE ALWAYS BEEN PATHETICALLY IN LOVE
WITH MY MOTHER." SHE TALKS ABOUT TRYING AGAIN AND AGAIN TO GET HER
MOTHER TO BE REAL, TO BE CLEAR, AND TO TELL THE TRUTH WITH HER

That *I am pathetically in love with my mother*: in a sense it can't ever
have been less than obvious. Still that seems different from feeling
moved, or able, to frame the sentence. I'm only just trying to feel my
way into what it means to find myself saying this.

One thing, though: it seems clear that I've been in full flight from
this utterance for twenty-five years.

Of course it's embarrassing! Because I've seen myself as such a
firm oedipal conscientious objector. Yet I'm also reassured by the
solid, dumb ordinariness of the sense of this

place where at last I'm
free to make myself at home,
just nosing around.

Of course, too, all this is swirling in a million different ways
around the prospect of my folks' meeting with Shannon. I have layer
on layer of painful fantasies. Most simply, that Shannon will take my
parents' part against me. Or that *he'll* fall in love with my mother. (I do

remind myself that at fifty, he may not be in the habit of falling for women of seventy-two). About this fear he asks: "So you and I would be competing for her?"

"It goes both ways. What struck me more was that you'd love her instead of me."

"I guess I need to practice seeing it like that," he says, "I was looking forward to saying to you, afterward, 'I really ——'d your mother!' — and filling in the blank with something like *enjoyed*, or *got a kick outta*."

Another fear: he might learn to see me as a denatured copy of a true original. I have this habit of thinking of my family as an especially pungent ragoût, with all the different flavors melding, the various proteins twining together. To me it has a distinctive flavor, culture, language. "And when someone comes along and just meets me, a little ladleful out of the big pot, and notices they haven't encountered this flavor before, they think of it as Eve-flavor.

"But then I worry that when they came to perceive it as, not Eve-flavor, but Kosofsky-flavor, I could get to seem very diminished."

I guess that worry's not about rivalry or opposition—just your basic individuation.

Here's my worst fear, though: that *she'll* say something to me about *him*, something contemptuous, that will decathect me from him suddenly, hard, and completely. (A certain horrifyingly efficacious style of "zinger"—a style I try heroically, mostly successfully, to suppress—is suddenly legible to me as a carbon-copy legacy of my mom's.) It could happen! —much as I love Shannon, even as much as I mistrust my mother.

This particular danger seems to catch Shannon's attention in a different way from the others. Maybe it surprises him, but he sees the realism of it. We go on about zingers, and when I describe the dynamics that tend to surround them, he notes there will be a loss in seeing my folks separately, too: he won't get to see them interacting.

At one point he tells me *his* fantasy: taking his own

"snapshot of the three
of you. You looking all small
and pale, next to them."

———————

"Waking up, thinking of questions for you to ask my folks . . . And
then I thought, well of course I can ask them questions myself; what
would I like to know from them?

Something came to me
that really caught hold of my
imagination.

I wanted to ask,
'If you were taking a walk
in the neighborhood,

and you came upon
a cluster of little girls
playing, and one of

them was me as a
little girl—would you know me?
Would you stop and say,

That one is Evie
as a little girl? You're *Eve*
and you have come back!

Would you be that sure?"
What a sentimental and
cruel test it is!

> Likelier, for that
> matter, *they* would know me so
> surely, than I would."

We moot some good approaches and questions for my folks. Shannon suggests, "Were there needs you saw this kid as having that seemed hard or painful to attend to?"

I like this—it seems empathetic rather than suspicious. Shannon says, "Really, I feel a lot of empathy with them.

"I'm not sure if you can tell that," he's going on, "because so much of the time I'm trying to get you to formulate your case against them. But I seem to identify a lot with what it must have been like to be in their position.

"Do you think I need to say that to them?"

I've laid my head back against the couch. I'm talking as if I were not there at all. "Oh, no. I'm sure it'll come through if you just act like yourself. I hope it will license them—in something like the ways it's licensed me . . . I've certainly always assumed at some base level you've *got* to be on their side,"

> which of course I have,
> though his saying just that, just
> *now*—well, it's a jolt.

Pathetically in love: it feels big, like the path of an avalanche.

But also hopeful on a remarkable scale.

All last night, dreams of extraordinary powers. In one dream I could write a whole line just by looking at the computer screen in a particular way.

"Any idea . . . ?"

"Yes, it makes sense to me actually, to feel the possibility of great powers living here. I take it as real.

"My affect toward other women—it's been so paralyzed all these years, and I know, I think I've always known, that was because of my terrorized flight from hopeless feelings about my mother. I think in the dream, it came to me that I might not have to be seventy before figuring out whether I'm a dyke or not!

"(You see I'm still competing with my mom . . .)

"This room called 'being in love with mother,' this seems so like a real place. A place to enter into; look around;

> a place you can go
> away from, and when you go
> back to, it's still there.

One that looks different from different viewpoints. Where you can be in it and have different moods and feelings, but the furniture is still the same. With something like all three dimensions to it."

THREE HOURS TODAY; E's MOTHER, THEN HER FATHER, THEN E LATE IN THE DAY. THE STYLE OF THE PARENTS IS QUITE DIFFERENT. RITA IS ALWAYS MOVING; YOU ARE NEVER SURE IF YOU WILL GET A "REAL" ANSWER, OR A "CANNED" ONE, OR AN EVASION.

"I've never met anyone who moves around so much," he tells me, "not physically but in terms of where she *is* in the conversation. It made me think of the old *Starship Enterprise*. 'Yes, I think we're getting a radar fix—*no*, it's *gone*, no, I think we're getting closer . . . Sorry, sir, it's drifting—yes *here* it is . . .'"

SHE COMMUNICATES THE PROMISE OF SOMETHING INTERESTING AND REAL AND SOMEHOW EDIFYING, BUT DOES NOT RELIABLY DELIVER.

"But you got the sense of why it would feel really valuable," I insist, "to get access to her truth-telling mode? Why it would matter to somebody?"

"Oh, yes. That was *very* clear."

SHE IS QUITE BRIGHT, ERUDITE, AND CREATIVE.

   THE FATHER IS MUCH WARMER AND KINDER, BUT WITHOUT THE BRIGHT INCISIVENESS OF HIS WIFE. HIS TALK IS ALLUSIVE AND FRAGMENTED——DENSE AND SOMEHOW MELANCHOLY. HE IS UNABLE TO TALK JUST ABOUT E WITHOUT BRINGING IN THE OTHER TWO CHILDREN IN SOME CONNECTED WAY

> "like each sentence out
> of his mouth is a way of
> saying, You kids stand
>
> closer together
> so I can get all of you
> into the snapshot.

"But, as you say—a sweetness."

HE ALSO DWELLS ON THE LATER YEARS EVEN WHEN I TRY TO GET HIM TO TALK ABOUT THE EARLY ONES.

   RITA, IN CONTRAST, STAYS WITH THE PRE-TEEN YEARS. SHE PRESENTS A PIC-TURE OF A CHILD WHO SPRANG INTO BEING FULLY FORMED. SHE REALIZED EARLY THAT E WAS BRILLIANT AND, DENYING ANY INTIMIDATION BY OR TROU-BLE WITH THE BRILLIANCE, SAYS SHE WAS NOT AFRAID OF E AS LONG AS SHE WAS BIGGER THAN E . . . THEN SAYS THAT THAT DIDN'T LAST LONG.

Shannon says the sense of this kid being uncanny or a changeling was stronger than he could have pictured. He mentions several stories they both told, going way back to toddlerhood, that somehow all led to the same punch line: "and from then on we realized she was going to go her own way." Somehow as if any display of my agency was the same as a full-scale declaration of independence? As if the day I quit nursery school was the day I left for college.

"From what you say I almost wonder if they perceived me as a child at all—whether they had any ordinary enjoyment of me as a kid, or attention to me as one, or worries about me, that weren't organized around the supposed strangeness of this presence."

"I tried and tried to elicit stories like that," he says. "They just wouldn't come up with any. Was she cute? Did you have fun with her? Did she have trouble teething? No."

A long pause.

THROUGHOUT THE INTERVIEW SHE CASTS THINGS IN TERMS OF "AREN'T ALL FAMILIES" OR "MOST CHILDREN ARE." YET SHE IS CLEARLY VERY INVESTED IN THIS GIRL.

"Your mother," Shannon says, "really was taken with you from very early on. I don't mean that in an enthusiastic way necessarily. But she communicates that she had a thing about you. Whatever she says, I think you did scare her; but also fascinated her. She said she often was surprised to find herself talking with you about things she wouldn't talk about with a child."

"But she was interested in me as a child?"

"No. Or if she was, at least it didn't come through to me."

ANOTHER TRAIT IS HER USE OF "NOT SOMETHING ONE WOULD ASK, OR TALK ABOUT, OR MENTION" IN A NUMBER OF CONTEXTS. SHE ALWAYS WONDERED WHY E & HAL DIDN'T HAVE CHILDREN BUT WOULD NEVER ASK. ESPECIALLY IN THE AREA OF SEXUALITY SHE SAYS THAT THEY WERE NOT RESTRICTIVE (WE NEVER COVERED THE CHILDREN'S NAKEDNESS) BUT NOT PRONE TO TALK ABOUT IT. BUT THEN SAYS THAT HER STUDENTS HAVE COMMENTED TO HER ON THE AMOUNT OF SEXUAL ALLUSION IN HER TEACHING. THEN SAYS THAT ALL CHILDREN ARE SEXUALLY AWARE AND FEELING EARLY. SHE WAS AWARE OF E'S MASTURBATION BUT, OF COURSE, WOULD NEVER HAVE MENTIONED IT. THE FATHER IS "IN AWE OF" E RATHER THAN BEING AFRAID OF HER.

I TALK WITH E, TELLING HER ALL THIS FOR ALMOST THE WHOLE HOUR. SHE IS QUITE PLEASED AND RELIEVED THAT I SAW THE THINGS SHE HAS BEEN TELLING ME SHE EXPERIENCED. AFTER THE HOUR, I FEEL SOME DOWN. AS BEST I FORMULATE IT, IT IS THAT WELL, YES, IT REALLY WAS LIKE I THOUGHT IT WAS AND SO NOW WHAT. NO SECRETS TO UNCOVER. NOTHING TO FIND OUT TO MAKE IT BE DIFFERENT. WILL SEE IF E HAS ANY OF THIS REACTION.

My mother tells me, "I was impressed with Shannon, he seemed so professional and competent. I could tell

> just by the way he
> paced the hour, starting off with
> some comments designed

> to put me at ease;
> and I appreciated
> how he was leading

> 'imperceptibly'
> up to more difficult things
> as the time went on . . ."

That night, my folks have a chance to compare notes about their conversations with Shannon. My father remarks on a phrase they both found themselves using: something like,

> "Eve always knew what
> she knew, and knew she knew it.
>   Whether she was *right* . . ."

But over the weekend I get a chance to ask my mother, "Can you bear another psychohistory question? Would you tell me some about what it was like for you to have Nanny as a mother?"

I see her scanning the angles of this question—

what particular
damning judgments of herself
mightn't it entail?

Finally, generously, she doesn't second-guess it. "Mmm. *Pretty good*, I'd say. Certainly, she tried hard. Pretty good . . . *considering*."

"How's that?"

"Well, of course different people would give you different answers about any parent. For me, the hardest thing about Nanny was her very loud voice. You know that's not something it's easy for me to deal with, and I've developed a very different manner from that, myself. *That* was painful for me.

"Also Nanny was very certain in her judgments; she always knew she was right. She had a hasty temper and she would let you feel her anger."

"Though," Daddy adds, "she never held a grudge."

"No, that's very true, when her anger was over, it was over."

"She was an intensely intelligent woman," my mother is going on, "intensely, and she accomplished an amazing amount considering her lack of education—if she'd been educated, she's somebody who would have made a mark in the world."

I pipe up, "It's always been hard for me to imagine Nanny as the mother of babies. I remember when I was little, she used to terrify me—always threatening to *gobble me up* because I looked so *delicious*. As if irony and aggression were her only modes of affection. 'You have such rough *skin*! Such *disgustingly* rough skin! RRRrrrr!' It was years before I could decide whether she actually meant these things: I re-member explicitly telling myself she couldn't, because everyone else said I had really soft skin! And even then I found it alarming. Her voice was so raucous, her movements were so startling and abrupt. But was she like that with you too?"

Yes, my mother says, she was.

———————

There's a pair of us?
She refined to her quiet
by the long labor

of refusing her
mother's noisy and pointed
wit of the fishwife—

and her own relish
in it—I, the refusal
of a refusal—

———————

Refusals everywhere, these corrosive ones—

All the same, Shannon says, it's probably still true, my mother's style of nurture must have derived a fair amount from her own mother's trenchant, impatient one. He's struck by so much evidence of "don't ask, don't tell" among the Kosofskys—especially about pain, psychic or physical.

(I think of her heroic, near-psychotic, exasperating denials: of ever feeling any illness, weakness, or fatigue. Even weather. Given her own way, she'd wear shorts all winter.

Once she channeled for me what she said was Nanny's response to illness in their family. "There's no money for doctors, so *you feel fine.*" Nanny, abruptly denuded of her own family by the flu epidemic in 1919.)

Shannon conjures my long childhood terror at Nanny's noisy assaults. "I don't think you'd have been as scared if you'd been able to look at Mommy and see her responding differently. If she'd found them funnily affectionate, or felt anyways clear how to interpret them. Instead she probably went rigid herself with something like fright—or else just left the room, you alone with Nanny."

Also, though: my mother could have felt, early on, somehow that this odd child's presence embodied her own mother. Someone she'd find, at unpredictable moments, really alarming—

the both of us so
quick to be certain that we
knew what we did know.

The dangerous thing about being mistaken by my mother for her own, apparently all-powerful, mother was that she would fantasize me, too, to be competent, powerful, invulnerable.

Me, sobbing and sobbing. But saying,

Okay—my mouth wants
to say she couldn't believe
that, being a child,

I needed care and
attention. But the simple
truth is that I still

identify with
her enough not really to
believe it myself.

But I still have to tell Shannon about the beautiful-feeling dream I had this morning, shortly before waking. In the dream, Shannon was the proprietor of a store—a wonderful store—that stocked food, books, and objets d'art. The kind of place where you would stop in just to look at what was there, even if you weren't buying. I did so (and noted that the place had expanded, in fact); but Shannon greeted me with a distressed face, saying, "You know that little goddess statue you liked so much?"

Now, as it happened, I couldn't remember any particular goddess. I tried to visualize it—a little limestone Venus? Anyway, though I couldn't remember, I nodded recognizingly.

"Well," he said, "I'm afraid it's broken. Here, you can see . . ." And he showed me the place on the floor where a Mexican pottery

goddess (maybe a
virgin of Guadeloupe)
still lay in pieces.

"Oh, that's okay," I said in the dream, "I really don't mind at all. But it's so kind of you to worry that I would, to imagine and identify with my distress about it."

————

"I've had in mind the
conventional terms of the
family romance

where *they* think I'm just
their kid, but *I* know that I'm
really the exiled

daughter of the king
and queen of Mars. But this is
just the opposite!

Isn't it? Where they
are convinced that, for better
or worse, I come from

some other planet—
and it's *I* who don't know,
I who think to be

their own, peasant child,
to be one of them.—In fact
who longs to be so."

Shannon makes it sound as though they were apt to treat me as a kind of independent contractor living in the house—or ambassador of a neighboring principality, maybe.

"Do you think that's why their discipline always felt so cataclysmically raw to me?" I suddenly think to ask. "It's not that it was frequent, or especially brutal. But it's children who get spanked, not ambassadors. If I was used to all that inexplicable protocol, then it must have felt like the strangest assault on my dignity. Almost, my national dignity! Mustn't it?

Shannon likes this. "Even quite severe discipline," he says, "doesn't traumatize kids so very much as it did you. Most children do understand it as a form of care. It's arresting to them, but *enough* familiar,

it's cut from the same
fabric as the other kinds
of care they're used to."

TERRIFYING DREAM OF A FASCIST SOCIETY, ORGANIZED LIKE A SUMMER CAMP AROUND CALISTHENTICS AND AEROBICS. SOMEONE HAS COMMITTED AN IN-FRACTION OF THE RULES AND IS TO BE KILLED. EVERYONE IS FURIOUS BUT NO ONE KNOWS HOW NOT TO BE COMPLICIT——AT MOST THEY CAN CONTINUE TO DO THE AEROBICS WITH AN ANGRY ENERGY. THEN E IS WITH A GROUP GOING OFF INTO THE DESERT. THEY SEE A MAN WITH A BURLAP BAG OVER HIS HEAD BEING

PUSHED OUT INTO THE DESERT TO BE KILLED. AGAIN E FEELS THAT THEY ARE IN
SOME KIND OF COMPLICIT RELATIONSHIP TO THIS. //

The next morning,

> just waking—massive
> as having a stroke—come two
> realizations.

> "But," I tell Shannon,
> "like *Jeopardy!*, the trick here
> is in the question.

"Here's the question: how to relate young Eve's family situation, on
the one hand, to her personal/professional/political/academic en-
gagements over the past fifteen years, and specifically her relation to
queer stuff, on the other?"

"Yeah? I'm listening."

"Okay, in each case, imagine somebody who expends extortionate
amounts of energy trying to convince the members of some group
(not a particularly privileged group, not a high-status group, in fact a
clannish, defensive, stigmatized, but proud, and above all an interesting group) that she, too, is to be accepted as—and in fact, truly is—a
member of this group. A kid, a Kosofsky—or later, gay. But each time
it's in the face of some inherent, in fact obvious absurdity about the
claim."

"But," Shannon sensibly asks her, "why would she want to do that?"

"Well of course as a kid, because I have no choice about it. But then
as an adult because—what, because it 'feels right,' feels productive
and *true*, too. Oh, and of course by then, because it's what I'm used to
doing."

Only visibly
more preposterous this time,
now that I almost

know what it is that
I'm claiming or offering—
it's like a big dare,

also like a big
allegory about love.
Experimental.

And at least to me,
metamorphic (which is how
I recognize love).

It's as if I can now understand the ineffable happiness—and the fragility and depletion attaching to it, too—that goes, for me, with being accepted and loved (in my personal life, I mean) as an essential, central member of a queer family. Whose ideology, yes, I do a lot of the work of articulating, making new, making compelling to others.

In this small (but not quite circumscribable) context, yes, I can recognize others and be recognized in many aspects that don't, this time around, seem to denegate one another: as loving *and* bright, as included and constitutive, and not too scary . . .

While on a bigger gay-lesbian scene, what I've maybe helped happen (both for me and for the self-perception and group perception of some other people) is so much more partial, iffy, streaky, potentially upsetting, often thrilling, feeling completely risky—but it's a recognizable transformation of the same project: trying to convince this family I'm not the daughter of the king and queen of Mars.

———————

Next thing I see: it makes so much sense how this adult project of queer community resonates with my old need to "be my mother's therapist," to promote her turning into somebody less anxious and fuller.

"Yeah, I know—big duh, right?"

"Well," Shannon says consideringly, "ye-e-es . . ."

Especially, I mean, to the extent that her potential for being different, and happier, was visibly tied up with a lesbian possibility.

Because that lesbian component went in

two directions whose
double-vectoring now feels
so familiar and

(in a bizarre way)
so "comfortable" to me: first,
as having something

obscurely to do with
who *I* was, woman myself.
But at the same time

how much of what she
suffered was a deeply lodged
protest against a

life immobilized
in this nuclear scene of
caring for children?

So the girl child who
somewhere in the future makes
part of the scene—still

has to nonexist
if the beloved is to
materialize.

———————

Melodrama of
uncertain agency, called
"Bringing Out Momma."

———————

BACK TO THE FASCIST DREAM, THE SENSE OF THAT CRUSHING LAW THAT SHAT-
TERED PEOPLE'S AGENCY——ALSO IN THE DREAM THE SENSE OF THE PEOPLE'S
REBELLION ORGANIZING AND TRYING TO MOBILIZE BUT NOT BEING ABLE TO——
CAN VIEW THE DREAM NOT JUST AS ANXIOUS ALARM BUT AS GROWING EDGE,
SOMETHING TRYING TO COME INTO EXISTENCE. (?ANY OTHER PLACE FEELING
THIS?) YEAH, SEXUALITY——AND IN THE AREA OF STUFF ABOUT POLITICAL AND
ETHICAL COMMITMENTS. // MUST EARLY ON HAVE BEEN THE MOMENTS OF BE-
ING HAMMERED, SHATTERED——BORN TOO EARLY TO BE ABLE TO ORGANIZE
THINGS, BUT IT BEING MY JOB TO ORGANIZE THEM.

———————

A BIG FIGHT WITH P.: E SAYS SHE CAN'T/DOESN'T DO ANGER, JUST CRIES——
FINDS IT HARD TO TOLERATE EITHER BEING IN THE RIGHT OR IN THE
WRONG——HOW CAN A RELATIONSHIP BE SO WOUNDING AND SO LOVING——
CAN'T BEAR TO HAVE PEOPLE ANGRY AT / REPROACHING ME. ASSERTING SELF OR
PUTTING SELF FORTH IN A RELATIONSHIP RUNS THE RISK OF RUPTURING IT.
BOMB IN THE BOSOM.

———————

GARY DIED LAST NIGHT. WE SPEND MUCH OF THE HOUR TALKING ABOUT THE DEATH, GARY HIMSELF, AND E'S REACTION TO IT, WHICH IS MOSTLY SLOW REALIZATION SO FAR. TOWARD THE END WE RETURN TO SEX AND TALK ABOUT HOW HARD IT IS TO FOCUS ON THIS TOPIC. PART OF THAT IS THE FACT THAT, WHILE SEX IS A PRESENCE IN E'S LIFE IN MYRIAD WAYS, THESE WAYS ARE SO DISCONTINUOUS. THIS MAKES IT HARD FOR HER OR US TO FORM A COHERENT NARRATIVE UNDERSTANDING OF IT. E NOTES THAT ALL THE ELEMENTS OF IT WERE THERE IN HER EARLY ADOLESCENT YEARS BUT HAVE BECOME MORE FRAGMENTED—INSTEAD OF MORE INTEGRATED—IN THE ENSUING YEARS.

8

Vivid and frightening dream where I'm conveyed in the front seat of a bus or big van (no seat belts), going at a somewhat uncontrollable pace on a terrible road that's congested with others all driving like maniacs. It's almost cartoon-like, but scary. At one point the bus/truck behind ours bumped (fairly gently) into the back of ours—but no one took any notice. Then another one, which my father was driving, came close enough for me to say or gesture something (some fairly gentle but aggressive joke) to my father, which he either took or (I think this is right) just pretended, jokingly, to take umbrage at—but the joking pretense involved his pulling his red pickup truck abruptly out of the traffic (straight across several fast, congested lanes) to, on the road shoulder, U-turn it around and "jokingly" appear prepared to launch it at us . . .

"Us" = ??

Narrow arteries, swarming with

madly-driven trucks
branching at unexpected
dangerous junctures . . .

Bloodstream?
This, the night after Gary's death.

———————

STILL FEELING BAD. BAD IN THE MIDST OF ALL THE ISSUES OF LIFE AND DEATH THAT ARE GOING ON. WE TALK MORE ABOUT BEING ATTRACTED TO THE DYING AND THE DEAD, TAKING CARE OF THE DYING, IDENTIFICATION WITH THE DISEASE, SOME FEELING OF CAUSING THE ILLNESS OR DEATH BY ENGAGING WITH IT, ETC. E NOTES THAT SHE IS FEELING MORE RELAXED SOMEHOW ABOUT THERAPY, ABOUT WRITING DOWN OUR SESSIONS; THE FEELING THAT SHE DOES NOT HAVE TO DO ALL THE WORK OR KEEP TRACK OF JUST WHERE WE ARE OR WHAT WE ARE PURSUING. THAT SHE CAN LEAVE SOME OF THAT TO ME, IN A WAY SHE HAS NOT BEEN ABLE TO DO PREVIOUSLY. WE MOVE BACK TO TALKING ABOUT SEX BUT VEER OFF INTO SOME TALKING ABOUT HER SISTER AND UPCOMING VISIT. THIS DOES NOT SEEM AVOIDANT BUT AGAIN THAT WE CAN TALK ABOUT SOMETHING AND COME BACK TO THE IMPORTANT TOPIC.

———————

REASSURED BY OUR LAST SESSION; NOTICEABLY LESS ANXIOUS. NOTES THAT SHE WAS SURPRISED TO HEAR HERSELF SAYING THAT I SEEM TO SUPPORT OR VALIDATE HER MAGICAL THINKING. SHE SAYS THAT REFLECTING ON THIS SHE THINKS IT IS ACCURATE, AND THAT SHE HAS BENEFITTED FROM IT, BUT THAT SHE WOULD HAVE THOUGHT THAT SHE WANTED THE MOST ROCK-SOLID, UNMAGICAL KINDS OF THINGS ON WHICH TO RELY. SOME OF THIS COMES FROM THE "SPECIAL FARE FOR CHILDREN" KINDS OF EPISODES, MOTHER'S SPOTTY SENSE OF REALITY, BUT MORE IT SEEMS TO BE RELATED TO THE FEAR OF ABANDONMENT.

———————

A few hours with some of Gary's papers, which I'll be editing for publication: two-hundred-proof taste of what the coming months hold as I plunge into the vat of his unmakings. Including, intensely: abyssal, glazed-over boredom.

Not because his writing fails to astonish.

This kind of boredom doesn't mean no-cathexis: this kind, to me, means overstimulation, stimulation of wrong or dangerous kinds; hell; rape; dissolution. The kind of boring that's a penetration.

"Informed" by my studious father, unable to escape.

Christopher Bollas writes about an effect he calls "extractive introjection." My association: a father who'd "extract" the child's interest in a subject—steal it, in effect, in the service of his own need to experience interest—and in its place, inject me with what he was *dis*owning: depressive deadness of attention and interest. *My* eyes glazing.

His painful inability to attend at the same time to a person and a subject.

Process I always—I don't know why—associate with rape. But also (as, more a writer, I've become less a reader) with reading someone else's writing when I'm not in a position to stop and write about it.

Writing, then, as a defense against reading?

So, I'm telling Shannon, a summer full of one version and another of these heightened acts of possession, habitation, uncertain agency.

Shannon: "You'll be okay? I have to ask that out of simply caring for you."

I think so. My plan for the summer feels like a slow descent into madness,

> but part of the plan
> is that you'll keep me okay.
> Don't you think so?
>   "Yes."

SHE BRINGS UP THE BOLLAS CONCEPT OF INTROJECTIVE EXTRACTION (I NEED TO READ THIS) AS IT CLEARLY REMINDS HER OF HER FATHER AND HIS ABILITY TO SUCK THE VITALITY OF A TOPIC OUT OF HER IF SHE BROUGHT THE TOPIC TO

HIM. SHE REMEMBERS HER ONLY DEFENSE AS BEING THE INTERNAL RETREAT FROM A SITUATION WHICH SHE COULD NOT REALLY ESCAPE.—AT THE END I FEEL IMPELLED TO TELL HER ABOUT THE HUEY P. LONG BRIDGE.

He's been in New Orleans, and he tells me about driving across a bridge there, some kind of marvel of unlikely and spectacular engineering. Describing it, he says, "It provoked these two, almost instantaneous thoughts. First: 'This is the kind of thing that Eve would *never* be interested in.' And second: 'I'm really looking forward to telling her about it anyway.'"

I'm tickled that he'd taken the thought of me along with him—and of course, anything he tells me does interest. In my mind it's connected with his mentioning, before he left town, "I'm glad they'll be painting my office while I'm gone, but I'm going to miss that stain over the couch. It gives me something to stare at when patients are talking—and I like thinking that it's shaped like the *Starship Enterprise*,"

> which had surprised me
> into this fond, sensuous,
> big snort, like, "Oh, *you*—!

"Of course it does! Of course it just does!"

———

I ASK HER ABOUT MY TELLING HER ABOUT THE BRIDGE. THIS SEEMS TO HAVE IMPORTANT DIFFERENCES FROM THE INTERACTIONS WITH HER FATHER, PARTICULARLY IN HIS ABILITY TO TAKE OVER A TOPIC AND DEADEN IT FOR HER. WE TALK AROUND THIS FOR A WHILE. I MENTION THAT I THINK IT MARKED A CHANGE IN HOW I FEEL ABOUT HER.

"I was looking forward to making it so you *would* be interested in the bridge. Thinking about it later, I saw that all this signified some real shift in my relationship to you. I'm feeling something I rarely do about patients: that being really seen by you is something that matters to me. Not that I just get narcissistically recirculated back to myself through your eyes, which happens all the time—but that I'm changed to myself in some way as I see that you see me.

"But then I'm thinking, if this is something I like getting from you, it could have meant a lot to other people, too. You tell me it happens with the friends you love—and I believe it, though that's not a kind of friendship I've got much experience of. But I'm thinking specially of your father, all those scenes where your eyes glaze over with refusal of his information: I'm wondering whether he would come to those scenes hoping to obtain this kind of transformative attention from you—"

Too good a question
to get a yes or no (plus
I am still *breathless*)—

THEN E TELLS ME ABOUT A MEMORY WHICH HAS BEEN ON HER MIND. IT IS A MEMORY, AGE 7 OR 8, OF A PARTICULARLY TRAUMATIC DENTIST VISIT. THE ELEMENTS SEEM TO BE HER FEELING/BELIEVING THAT SHE AND THE DENTIST HAD AN UNDERSTANDING OR SOMETHING, THAT HE LIKED HER AND FOUND HER EXCEPTIONAL. HER EXPERIENCES WITH HIM WERE RELATIVELY PAIN-FREE (DESPITE NO NOVOCAIN) UNTIL ONE DAY SHE HAD SEVERAL FILLINGS DONE IN ONE AFTERNOON AND IT WAS EXHAUSTING AND VERY PAINFUL, AND SHE WAS UNABLE TO GET AWAY, AND PERHAPS UNABLE TO PROTEST—STUCK THERE WHERE SHE HAD GONE SO WILLINGLY. THIS SEEMS TO BE SIMILAR TO A CONCEPT OF RAPE TO HER, SOME SIMILAR TO THE ABOVE EPISODES WITH HER FATHER, AND SIMILAR TO HER MASOCHISTIC FANTASIES. ANOTHER IMPORTANT PART IS THAT SOMEHOW THIS IS HER 'FAULT' (?) IN THE SENSE OF HAVING THOUGHT THINGS WERE OTHERWISE WITH THE DENTIST, OR PRESUMING ON AN ATTRACTION/UNDERSTANDING BETWEEN THEM WHICH HE WAS FINALLY FREE TO IGNORE AND DID.

TALKS ABOUT FINDING THE PIECING TOGETHER OF THINGS ABOUT HER CHILD-
HOOD LESS ENGAGING THAN TALKING ABOUT THE SEXUAL FANTASIES OR AT-
TENDING TO WHAT IS GOING ON BETWEEN US THAT SHE CALLS THE TRANSFER-
ENTIAL ASPECTS OF THE THERAPY. BOTH OF US NOTE THAT WE HAVE BEEN NOT
TALKING ABOUT THE SEXUAL FANTASIES, THAT E HAS BEEN BRINGING IN
VIGNETTES OF HER EXPERIENCE TO RELATE INSTEAD. SHE NOTES THAT SHE IS
ANXIOUS AT THE PROSPECT OF NOT HAVING SOMETHING TO TALK ABOUT. AS WE
BOTH SAY WE WILL TALK MORE ABOUT THIS ON FRI. E BECOMES ANXIOUS WITH-
OUT KNOWING WHY.

HAD REAL DENTIST APPT. EARLIER TODAY, WENT RELATIVELY WELL IN THE PRES-
ENT, ALTHOUGH SOME OF THE SYMPTOMS OF THE DENTIST PHOBIA CAME BACK
EVEN WITH TWO VALIUM; WAS ABLE TO TELL THE HYGIENIST AND GET DENTIST
TO NUMB THE MOUTH. THIS NOTES THAT THE FOCUS OF THE FEAR SEEMS TO BE
PAIN WHICH IS EXPECTED BUT YOU DON'T KNOW WHEN AND YOU CANNOT PRE-
PARE YOURSELF FOR IT. NEITHER I NOR E CAN THINK OF AN ANALOGOUS PAIN,
AND THE SCENE OF SPANKING DOES NOT SEEM TO BE RELEVANT. SHE IS STILL
SOME SHAKEN FROM THE REEXPERIENCING OF THE CHILDHOOD HELPLESS-
NESS. ALSO, HAD BEEN THINKING ABOUT MY COMMENT THAT SHE DWELLS ON
THINGS.

"I think this accounts for a big part of the sheer pleasure I get from
therapy. Of course a lot of it is simply liking you, but also a lot of the
just-plain-sweetness of the thing is that I always feel there's a fresh
supply of narrative coming my way to brood over. And then there's the
thing"—

I have trouble formulating this; the next few sentences are halt-
ingly assembled. "You know, when I start telling you something by
saying, 'I was thinking about what you said about . . . ,' it always gives
me pleasure to say that, to let you know that I was brooding on your
words. And I think the pleasure is . . . well, I know how much I love it
when *you* say 'I was thinking about what you said about . . . ' It's
somehow as though the part of you that's in me will be able to nour-

ish the part of me that's in you, or—something—I don't know how to put it. But that there's some circuit of reciprocity between these holding relations: your ability to hold me inside you, and mine to hold you inside me."

It goes back to things we've talked about before, about object permanence. It seems clear I must have had this exciting pleasure, at least intermittently, as a child.

REFLECTING, E REALIZES THAT SHE HAS FELT DIFFERENT SINCE MY HUEY LONG COMMENTS THAT SOMETHING HAD CHANGED IN THE RELATIONSHIP BETWEEN US. SHE HAS HAD MULTIPLE REACTIONS TO THIS. SHE HAS BEEN AFRAID THAT IN MY GETTING THINGS FROM HER, THAT I WILL STOP BEING THERE FOR HER NEEDS. SHE HAS BEEN AFRAID THAT IF SHE DOES NOT CONTINUE TO BE WHATEVER SHE IS IMAGINING BEING FOR ME THAT I WILL LOSE INTEREST OR BE ANGRY WITH HER. SHE HAS BEEN PLEASED THAT SHE IS ABLE TO BE WHATEVER FOR ME—WHICH SHE SEES SOME AS THE MAKING SMARTER PROJECT. SHE HAS REPLAYED THE DENTIST SCENARIO WITH THE PRESUMPTUOUS GIRL THINKING THERE WAS AN UNDERSTANDING. SHE NOTES THAT SLOWLY OVER TIME SHE HAS MOVED FROM VALUING MOST MY LISTENING FACE AND THE ENVIRONMENT IT MADE FOR HER, TO ACTUALLY VALUING ME AND WHAT I SAY AS WELL. THIS MOVES HER FROM THE POSITION OF HAVING TO DO ALL THE WORK, FIGURE OUT ALL THE ANSWERS, TO A POSITION WHERE SHE MIGHT FIND SOME HELP OR REAL ASSISTANCE.

IN RETROSPECT, SEVERAL ELEMENTS PLAYED INTO THIS DAY'S SESSION. I HAD HAD AN ANXIETY PROVOKING CONVERSATION WITH G. [ANOTHER THERAPIST IN THE PRACTICE] JUST BEFORE SEEING E AND LET HER KNOW I WAS UPSET. SHE HEARD IT AS MY HAVING TROUBLE WITH ANOTHER OF THOSE "PUSHY WOMEN" AND I SAID IN THE MIDST OF THIS THAT MY IMPULSE WAS TO WANT NEVER TO TALK TO G. AGAIN. FURTHER, I HAD BEEN CONCERNED AT THE CHANGE E TALKED ABOUT LAST HOUR, NOT KNOWING WHAT IT MEANT OR PORTENDED. IN

CONSEQUENCE, I WAS MORE RESERVED AND UNFOCUSED WITH HER THIS HOUR. THIS PANICKED HER. SHE GOT BOTH FRIGHTENED AND QUITE ANGRY WITH ME SPECIFICALLY FOR BEING VAGUE AND FUZZY. UPSETTING SESSION FOR BOTH OF US.

WE TALK ABOUT THE ABOVE; BOTH OF US HAVE ROUGHLY THE SAME PERSPECTIVE ON IT. AND WITH ME BACK NOT SO VAGUE THINGS GO MUCH SMOOTHER. INCIDENTALLY, E IS QUITE PLEASED THAT SHE COULD GET ANGRY WITH ME— ALWAYS DIFFICULT FOR HER TO FEEL AND EXPRESS ANGER AND SHE HAD WONDERED IF SHE WOULD BE ABLE TO EXPRESS IT TO ME. THE GLAZED LOOK SHE SAW IN MY EYES IS HER FATHER, RATHER THAN HER MOTHER.

LATE MAKING NOTES ON THIS SESSION—LITTLE MEMORY. SOMETHING OF THE CALM AFTER THE STORM OF THE LAST COUPLE OF SESSIONS. THIS PLUS MORE AS WE RETURN TO HER FATHER. SHE HAD SAID LAST HOUR THAT SHE HAD HER FATHER'S BODY, A STATEMENT WHICH HAD SURPRISED ME AS I HAD NOT THOUGHT OF HER BODY IN THIS WAY; AND A STATEMENT WHICH SURPRISED HER IN ITS DEFINITENESS. SHE BRINGS IN PICTURES OF HERSELF AND HER FATHER. SHE DOES HAVE HIS BODY (LARGE SQUARE FRAME) AS CONTRASTED WITH HER MOTHER.

SHE TELLS ME HER MOTHER'S DENTIST STORY. ASKED, HER MOTHER SAYS SHE DID NOT NOTICE THAT THERE HAD BEEN ANY PROBLEM BETWEEN E AND THE DENTIST. E ASKS, WHY WASN'T I GETTING NOVOCAIN? MOTHER SAYS THIS PROBABLY HAPPENED BECAUSE THE DENTIST ASKED E IF SHE WANTED "A NEEDLE" AND E REFUSED (ANOTHER DECLARATION OF INDEPENDENCE, AGE 8). MOTHER THEN TELLS A STORY OF HER OWN: SHE WAS BEING HURT IN THE DENTIST'S CHAIR AND THE DENTIST FINALLY NOTICING AND BEING TOUCHED AND TAK-

ING HER IN HIS ARMS, CRYING AND COMFORTING HER; THEN THAT HE LATER
LEFT THE PROFESSION. !!!

———————

Writing to Tim: I see, looking back, that a lot of the sense of con-
straint, for me, in the last several sessions actually, and despite the air-
clearing, has had to do with my sense of needing to perform some
"delicate" and stabilizing management of the Fact of (or what I took to
be the Fact of) Shannon's avowal of my functioning as something of a
transformational object for him as he also does for me. ("Transf. obj."
is Bollas again.) The not unfamiliar unsettlements, let me see, could
probably be classified under the headings, *Is he in love with me??* Does
that mean I've *won?* Would it mean I've *lost?* If I am truly *exceptional
among his patients*, how can I let him know that (a) I *know this*, and (b)
I nonetheless will never presume on it? At the same time, is it good
for me to feel as if I am being allowed to take some responsibility for
him, for recognizing and perceiving him, making him smarter, etc.?
Will I be able to stop doing this? (Since it's generally a lot easier for me
to take responsibility for somebody else's self-perception than for becoming visible to myself.) There's some level at which "*it* (some dis-
tinction, some 'precocious' recognition or responsibility)

> makes me happy, but
> is it good for me? *Ought* they
> to give this to me?"

is a deeply familiar question from a time I didn't feel sure I could
guard my own safety. I'd sure be interested in remembering why.

———————

Again to Tim, after my sleepless night and his interested e-mail response:

Oh, right, I keep forgetting, for lots and lots of people in the world, the notion of "falling in love" has (of all things) sexual connotations. No, that's not what I think is happening. For me, what falling in love means is different. It's a matter of suddenly, globally, "knowing" that another person represents your only access to some vitally

transmissible truth
or radiantly heightened
mode of perception,

and that if you lose the thread of this intimacy, both your soul and your whole world might subsist forever in some desert-like state of onto-logical impoverishment.

For me the sex comes in, I guess, in an instrumental way, if it does at all. Like, it's one possible avenue of intimacy—but if you have other good ones, like therapy, then I can never remember why somebody'd bother with sex.

Oh, and thank you for saying "Who is Shannon not to fall in love with you?"!

———————

E BEGINS ANXIOUSLY TODAY SAYING SHE AWOKE THIS MORNING AFRAID THAT I WOULD THROW HER OUT OF THERAPY. AS WE GO OVER THIS, SHE HAS BEEN AFRAID THAT OVER THE LAST THREE WEEKS SINCE SHE WAS ANGRY WITH ME, AND SINCE SHE WAS LETTING HERSELF BE BRIGHT AND SUCCESSFUL AND A SUR-PLUS WITH ME, THAT I HAD SEEMED UNABLE TO FOCUS SHARPLY ESPECIALLY ON TRANSFERENTIAL ISSUES. SHE BELIEVED THAT I HAD DECIDED THAT THIS AVOIDANCE WAS THE BETTER THERAPY POSITION AS A WAY OF DEALING WITH MY COUNTERTRANSFERENCE. SHE FEARED THAT I WAS AFRAID I WOULD FALL IN LOVE WITH HER, OR ALREADY HAD DONE SO, AND THAT I WOULD DECIDE THIS WASN'T GOOD (FOR HER) (FOR ME) AND THROW HER OUT OF THERAPY. IN RE-SPONSE, AS WE HAD TALKED OVER THE LAST WEEK OR SO, SHE HAD BEEN TRYING AND TRYING TO TALK ABOUT THE HERE AND NOW AND I HAD BEEN CONSIS-TENTLY INTERPRETING THIS BACK TO CHILDHOOD. SHE EXPERIENCED THIS AS

A CONFLICT IN WHICH SHE HAD TO PASSIVELY GIVE IN TO WHAT I WANTED
TO TALK ABOUT. // AS WE TALK I CLARIFY THAT THIS HAS NOT QUITE BEEN THE
CASE AND THAT I SEE HER AS BEING ABLE TO ATTEND JUST FINE TO HERSELF
AND SOMEONE ELSE TOO, AND THAT BESIDES I WOULD NOT THROW HER OUT
OF THERAPY.

When I ask him directly, abruptly, shyly, late in the session, "You
wouldn't kick me out, would you?"—there's a big smile for me, and
"No-o-o-o-o!" in an incredulous, somewhat tender whinny.

The nice thing is I don't wind up feeling unloved . . . Shannon's
sunny, resilient, lightly slobbish ways are great in this kind of fine-
honed high-hysterical crunch. At one point I marvel, looking back,
"But it seemed like such a seamless and inexorable braid of fatal in-
ferences!"

He responds with high interest, "I feel like, 'Gee, we don't have
one of those at our house—how does it work?'"

When he asks me how it started, the fantasmatic chain that had
led to this awful sense of impasse, I try for a long time to think what
to say, then just: "You were there for all of it; I don't know what else to
say!"

But then some things occur to me I know he wouldn't have been
aware of: like my sense of "free-floating remediation," especially for
possessing such a great wealth of good friendships and for his apparently not feeling well-friended in general. This is hard for me to make
myself say—it seems so pitiable, not to have plenty of good friends—
but he nods in slightly mournful recognition; he knows what I'm talking about.

Also the way some of my sadistic impulses, sadistic or just trenchant, manifested in the big fights we had or even just some regular language about him—the way that tends to boomerang around with a
sense of injury to him, a sense of his lackingness or neediness, a sense
of my plenitude, a sense of needing to spend my substance on these
interminable remediations . . .

"So you feel," he says, "as though just showing off—I don't mean
showing off ostentatiously" (he makes a theatrical gesture), "but just

showing" (a modest but wide opening-an-accordion gesture)—"You feel as though just the display of some aspect of you that involves this wealth and plenitude, like your good friendships, is going to hurt me, or someone, in a way that will involve you in an endless hemorrhage of self to make up for . . ."

"Yeah. Apparently."

About him, in my fantasy, about my parents

maybe here's the real
question: Can I turn them into who I need them

to be in order
to nurture me properly,
without "tempting" them

into something that
would destroy *me*—destroy *them*—
and destroy the scene

of their nurturance
for good?
　　　　With Shannon, maybe
one answer is, Yes.

————

TALKS SOME MORE ABOUT HER SEXUAL FANTASIES. SHE FINDS IT PLEASURABLE/
SATISFYING TO AGAIN BE THINKING ABOUT THESE AS SHE HAS NOT FOR SOME
TIME, ESP FROM THE PERSPECTIVE OF A CHILD.

But, he asks me, why not for some time?

He knows I've written and thought about all this, but not for a decade.

These motifs, I tell him—and the hours-long bouts of sexual reverie that used to accompany them—they've tailed off a lot in the past few years.

Partly it's menopause.

Also, though, the fortuitous meeting of the particular talents I've had on offer, with the snowballing of gay-lesbian studies, has given me a big, additional reason for being shy about my actual sexuality (if this even is one). Since it makes such a bad fit—and it's been so much easier just to put other people's queer sexuality in the place of my own, the place where, anyway, so much of my identification, passion, and thinking have always lived.

"But why is all this *so* hard to talk about? Even with me?"

So I try to describe the two magnetic fields I have to cross in trying to do it. On the one hand, since all the thematics and even particular words and phrases are sexual hot spots, I worry about getting turned on and short-circuiting the whole thing. While on the other, there's the teeth-grinding embarrassment of how discontinuous this fantasy material seems from any aspect of my life that I'm comfortable talking about or embodying.

"And moving between these isn't made any easier, I promise, by the fact that sexiness and embarrassment are two things that won't ever stay separate for me."

Actually, the space of talking to Shannon may be the best so far for keeping both arousal and embarrassment at just enough of a distance that I maybe can tread a line between. I tell him so: the first acknowledgment that it's *exciting* to me to talk about this with him.

"But in these fantasies," Shannon says, "isn't the emphasis more on acts and organs than words and phrases?"

"*You* know how fantasy works," I retort airily. But does he? I try my best. "It's like a closed room with all the air sucked out of it—hence, no gravity—and just a few, diverse objects tumbling around together. And the objects could be anything; they're in all different registers. Some of them, yes, would be words and phrases, some of them acts, organs, angles . . . And what makes them add up to 'fantasy' is that there isn't a stable context for them, or a stable place to identify, or anything."

"Like . . . ?" he asks. Or maybe, "Phrases like . . . ?" A long pause while I consider what I can say.

"Well, like when I told you about the nurse trying to get blood, in the room with the beds and the curtains, and then hearing somebody whisper, 'Spread your legs'? Now that would be a phrase that could turn up anywhere in my fantasies. Something like that.

"And other elements in the vacuum room? Well, say—particular organs—butts, assholes, women's genitals. And then, another element will always be some kind of institutional or quasi-institutional setting: a school, an institute, a hierarchy, something like that.

"Another kind of element would be a relation of witness or overhearing: somebody watching, the door left ajar, someone overhearing with pity, someone spying with malice, on the scene of punishment.

"An element will always be some speech or action of coerced consent from the person being punished. And that's a place where my identification is, for the moment, always glued to that person: just there, at that fold of wanting to withhold consent but being forced to perform it.

"Certain rhythms, too, might count as an element—spanking rhythms most obviously. Waiting—waiting with dread. I think those are the main things, at least the main kinds of things in that room."

I'm proud of producing this account. It seems like a viable mix of concrete and abstract, for this context, today anyway. (All this time, a lot of silent negotiation about what can be said with Shannon's and my eyes meeting, and what requires one or the other, or both, to throw our gaze to another corner of the room—at least to unfocus our pupils. But that, we can do.)

Eventually he notes, "I'm getting a warm, 'at-home,' pleasurable affect from you as you talk about this. Can you tell? It's real different from the anxious way you'd talk about actual childhood scenes of punishment, waiting, masturbation."

I say, with just

a little play of
impatience, "Well, it *is* my
sexuality—

yes, pleasure accompanies it." Yes, I add later, I do have the sense of a machine humming along that I can get energies from.

Near the end of the hour, a demon overtakes me and volunteers that it might even be possible to construct a chronology of these fantasies over the many years.

———————

WE MOVE TO SPANKING AS THE INTRO TO SEX. SHE HAS NO MEMORIES SPECIFI-
CALLY OF BEING SPANKED BUT CAN RESONATE TO THE SCENE OF HAVING TO
WAIT TILL FATHER COMES HOME TO BE SPANKED AND THERE BEING SOME RIT-
UAL OF COERCED CONSENT WITH HER HAVING TO PULL DOWN HER PANTS AND
BE OVER HER FATHER'S LAP. SHE CAN IMAGINE TRYING TO ARGUE WITH THE
PUNISHMENT, NOT UNDERSTANDING IT, SPENDING SOME TIME WHILE WAITING
FOR HIS RETURN MASTURBATING. IT IS UNCLEAR HOW THIS MIGHT HAVE BE-
COME WOVEN INTO THE SADO-MASOCHISTIC FANTASIES.

Trying to reconstruct the scene of spanking from all its traces in my narrative life. My sister says it was Daddy who spanked—all these years I'd never been able to remember who. But both parents must have been present, at least a lot of the time—I infer this from having not known for so long, but also from how instantly threat and rage get triggered in me (or in another register, porn excitement) by the exchange of language between adults about punishing children.

Similarly the mix of prurience and self-righteousness in adult language; the disavowed excitement.

Shannon is struck by the gaps that seemed to lurk in this narrative: between the deed and punishment; between the moment of parental anger and the moment of spanking. The productivity of those gaps! And near certainty that, in them, I generated attempts to argue my way out of being punished—argued "as one person to another," not as a kid to adults. Maybe this succeeded once or twice?

Or never.

Oh, but I'm a slow learner as far as giving up hope for getting things articulated, properly, *this time*. Shannon and I discuss the likely exacerbating effects of my attempts: instead of not being punished, would it be as if I were being punished, in this way, *as an adult*?

"You're not too old to
be spanked, you know"—a phrase
rank with its bad faith.

I say to Shannon, even if spanking hadn't gotten eroticized for me long before this phrase appeared (though I'm sure it had), this would have done it, wouldn't it?

Curious where there is to go from here.

Curious that I'm willing or able to focus on this instead of (in place of? in any relation to? I can't tell) the loss of Gary, unaddressed still in the reservoir of feelings. Somehow it's as if the level of pain or grrrindingness in talking about this stuff seems more bearable in the face of the huge, unaddressed loss.

Really don't know why.
Do feel inclined to use it,
push on, if I can.

———

HISTORY OF SEXUAL FANTASIES PROJECT——REALLY GOT RIGHT BACK INTO THE SEXUAL EXCITEMENT, FUN, ENJOYMENT, ETC., OF CONSTRUCTING THEM——BUT ALSO THE POINT OF VIEW FROM WHICH THEY ARE BORING, BANAL, STEREO-TYPIC——AND THERE IS THE SENSE OF PRIDE——ME TRYING, EARLY, TO MAKE A PLACE FOR MALE SEXUALITY AND GENITALIA IN MY PSYCHE. TRIED BUT DIDN'T GET TOO INTERESTED IN THAT. I ASK ABOUT THE BANAL VIEW SAYING I AM NOT SURE WHAT SHE IS SAYING AS THEY SEEM INTERESTING AND EXCITING TO ME, NOT BORING, BANAL.

Meanwhile, outside/around therapy, I've been enjoying a sensual reality and sense of possibility that I can't remember when I've felt before. I mean, of the reality of my own body. Which seems both the most natural thing in the world, and quite unaccountable (when I think of the actual content of these fantasies).

Also most strange is reading *Middlemarch* for school—loving it this time around—feeling at my very most Victorian-heroine-identified, ardent, longing, ethically pure and searching and demanding, etc., etc.—pouring all this out toward my classes—and at the same time, feeling so beautifully half-lost in this world of quite unintermitted brutality and punishment.

This time: George Eliot and the masturbating girl?

———

TALKS ABOUT THE WHOLE ISSUE OF BEING FAT BEING AT THE BOTTOM OF MANY OF THE SEXUAL FANTASIES——HER WAY OF SQUEEZING SOME SWEETNESS OUT OF THE ONGOING PAIN OF BEING UNACCEPTABLE. THAT THIS MAY BE MORE BASIC THAN THE ANAL-CENTEREDNESS OF THE FANTASIES. A WAY OF GIVING SOME SHAPE THAT SHE CAN WRAP HER MIND AROUND TO THE AMORPHOUS VIOLENCE. TALKS TOO ABOUT ALL OF THE FACETS EVOKED BY GIVING THESE FANTASIES TO ME——FEARS THAT I WILL BE BORED, FEARS I WILL BE TOO INTERESTED, THAT I WILL RESPOND TO THEM AS MYSELF INSTEAD OF RESPONDING TO THEM AS HER, THAT IT WILL BE WASTING HER TIME TRYING TO GET ME INTERESTED SEXUALLY IN SOMETHING THAT DOESN'T INTEREST ME, THAT THESE HAVE BEEN SO LONG IMPACTED THAT SHE WONDERS IF SHE CAN OPEN THEM OUT AND STILL BE LOVED, THAT IT WILL INTRODUCE A TONE OF GRINDING, BORING HARD WORK INTO THERAPY THAT HAS BEEN EXCITING AND ENJOYABLE . . .

———

"Remember when you asked for some specific phrases from the fantasy room—and after that long pause, I invoked the whole story of the nurse getting blood, and 'spread your legs,' and I said that was a phrase I recognized from my fantasies?

"Well, of course that was a real example. But the reason I chose that one is that it seemed to solve the problem of how I could answer your question truthfully, but in a way that would be—I don't know—swaddled up in enough narrative stuff that I could bear to say it.

"I mean, if I'd answered with perfect truth, I don't think the most indicative phrase would even have been 'spread your legs' but probably, like, 'pull down your pants.' But I didn't have a story to embed that in, at the moment, so I couldn't say it."

(Brightening up.) "But
of course, now I do, so I
can!"

"And so you do."

———————

SHE IS FEELING THAT I MUST NOT WANT TO TALK ABOUT HER SEXUAL FAN-
TASIES. I AM NOT AWARE OF TRYING TO AVOID THESE BUT SHE IS WORRIED THAT
I AM. AS WE TALK OVER THIS SHE BECOMES AWARE THAT SHE IS COUNTING ON
ME TO KEEP THE QUESTION OF WHETHER SHE WAS SEXUALLY ABUSED ALIVE BE-
CAUSE SHE DOES NOT FEEL SHE CAN RAISE IT HERSELF. SHE WANTS IT KEPT
ALIVE BECAUSE SHE VERY MUCH WANTS TO HAVE AN EXPLANATION FOR WHY
SHE IS THE WAY SHE IS, ESPECIALLY IN THE SEXUAL AREA BUT ALSO IN THE AREA
OF BEING DEPRESSED. SHE IS SURPRISED THAT SHE HAS BEEN USING ME FOR
THIS PURPOSE.

—Because if we've long agreed on one thing, it's not to be overtaken by an ambient discourse in which "sexual abuse" offers every answer to every question. And besides the lack of good suspects in my history, there's not the right *scale* of damage, it finally seems.

But somehow I still
can't let go the gravity
of Shannon's witness—

BEGINS BY BEING UPSET THAT SHE WAS SO MUCH LESS THAN HONEST WITH
HERSELF IN PROJECTING ONTO ME THE RESPONSIBILITY FOR KEEPING THE
ABUSE QUESTION ALIVE. THIS TIES IN WITH ME AS THE MAN PASSING BY THE
DOOR. SHE MOVES TO TELLING ME MORE OF ONE OF HER FANTASIES—THE MAN
FROM UNCLE. IN THIS THE POSITION OF COERCED CONSENT IS SPLIT BETWEEN
THE TWO MEN WHO MUST WATCH EACH OTHER TORTURED AND CAN STOP IT BY
TELLING THE SECRET THEY MUST NOT TELL. THE ENDING BACK AT HEADQUAR-
TERS WHERE THEY ARE WELCOMED AND PUNISHED LOVINGLY IS NOTABLE.

Somehow Shannon figures out a way of listening to fantasy that leaves
me feeling I've revisited it accompanied by a friend. He admires and
enjoys the elegance of the thing (this one is a densely overdetermined
and in that way *beautiful* fantasy).

He says, "I can see how a fantasy like this would be satisfying over
a period of years. Like art. You can turn it around and around."

He says, toward the end of the hour, "And that part where the one
guy is tapping on the stick in the other guy's ass—I *like* that detail, I
can feel it." And: "Are the other fantasies like this one?" he asks, as if
welcomingly.

With my sheepish pride I admit, "There are only a handful or two
where you can walk from room to room like this and look around. Some
of them are much thinner: just a few phrases, an image, an angle."

He asks some other questions that interest me. Do I empathetically experience the torture? Yes.

Do I have a mental picture of the torturers? Not at all; in most of
the fantasies, he/they are completely sketchy. The couple of excep-
tions (I never noticed this!) involve women who punish. In one case
clearly me; in another case clearly (not explicitly) my mother. Otherwise, this figure is left blank.

The *Man from UNCLE* fantasy ends with the Ilya Kuryakin char-
acter actually castrated—then back at UNCLE, punished again, this
time for giving away the crucial secret. How, Shannon asks, in my
imagination does he feel at the end of the fantasy?

"Great!" I rather surprise myself by announcing. "Well, oh, not exactly great—completely flattened, as a matter of fact; all is lost; blank. But he's cemented into this warm space of loss and punishment; seamlessly married to his work and the organization, as I guess he's always longed to be. And he's succeeded in declaring his love for Napoleon, and done it in a way that Napoleon has to be grateful for and pitying of. It just feels perfect."

The funny thing is that I think by now the sense of "perfect" is also radiating from my body language and voice. I wonder what age Shannon perceives me as being? I mean, I wonder what age I am?

Later, as other old fantasies are suddenly swarming to mind, there's a bolting panic about the thought of telling them—and beneath it a

stirring swell of the
likely *fun* of doing so.
Quite unexpected.

————

IF I TAKE THE KNOT OF COERCED CONSENT AND ASK WHAT PROBLEMS DOES THAT CONDENSE OR SOLVE OR DEFER? VARIED——FROM NO CONSENT, HAVING THINGS DONE TO YOU, TO RAW DEMAND. ONE OLD FANTASY IS A DISCIPLINARY INSTITUTION WHERE PEOPLE GET TAKEN TO GET PUNISHED, SPECTATORS PAY TO WATCH. CATCH WAS THAT SPECTATORS WOULD VOTE EACH TIME TO LET ONE PERSON OFF, SO EACH PERSON TO BE PUNISHED HAD TO GIVE A SPEECH TO ELICIT SYMPATHY——BUT THE SPEECH HAD TO BE VERY SPECIFIC, NUMBER OF COMPULSORY PHRASES, HAD TO SAY HOW THEY WERE TO BE PUNISHED IN FORMULAIC WORDS AND HOW PAINFUL/HUMILIATING IT WOULD BE——SO THE MORE HURTFUL AND HUMILIATING WOULD MAKE THE AUDIENCE WANT TO SEE IT MORE, BUT YOU HAD TO MAKE IT H&H ENOUGH TO GET THE SYMPATHY TO GET LET OFF. I ADMIRE HOW MANY FIERCE ENERGIES ARE IN THAT AND HOW IMMOBILIZED THEY ARE BY THE CROSS CONSTRAINTS.——MAY HAVE REMEMBERED THE ORIGINAL MOMENT OF COERCED CONSENT——BOOK OF S. ALEICHEM SHORT STO-

RIES PARENTS HAD, ONE I READ ABOUT AGE 7–8——LITTLE BOY TALKING ABOUT
A CRUEL SCHOOLMASTER WHO WOULD MAKE US PULL UP OUR OWN SHIRTS TO
BE WHIPPED——DON'T KNOW IF IT GRABBED ME BECAUSE OF FINDING IN WRIT-
ING SOMETHING ALREADY IN MY FANTASIES OR WHETHER IT WAS A NEW
THING.——BRUTE FORCE ON ONE END OF THE CONTINUUM AND MY PLEASURE
AT THE OTHER.

———

PRESENTATION OF GARY'S MATERIAL AT TWO CONFERENCES OVER THE WEEKEND
REMINDS E THAT SHE IS THE WRONG PERSON TO BE PROMOTING THIS MATERIAL.
IT IS ABOUT AND BY A BLACK MAN AND SHE IS WHITE; HE IS GAY AND SHE IS NOT;
THE MATERIAL HAS CONSIDERABLE ANGRY RACIAL MATERIAL AS WELL AS BEING
ABOUT SEX AND ABOUT MASTER-SLAVE SEXUAL RELATIONSHIPS; FINALLY THERE IS
A LONG "COLONIAL" HISTORY OF WHITE WOMEN PATRONIZING BLACK WRITERS.
HOWEVER, SHE FEELS SHE HAS ALWAYS BEEN THE WRONG PERSON TO DO THINGS
SHE HAS DONE PROFESSIONALLY AND HAS SOME INVESTMENT IN MAKING THAT
WORK, OR IN DEMONSTRATING THE INTEREST OF THAT BORDER-CROSSING POSI-
TION. SHE IDENTIFIES IT AS "KOSOFSKY" IN SOME WAY AND RELISHES THE AC-
COMPLISHMENT.——TOWARD THE END OF THE HOUR SHE TALKS ABOUT A FRIEND
WHOSE THERAPIST HAS "PUT HER ON THE COUCH." SHE HAS A CURIOSITY ABOUT
TRYING OUT THIS ARRANGEMENT——TO SEE WHAT THE S/M CONNOTATIONS ARE,
TO SEE WHAT IT DOES TO THE THERAPEUTIC BOND, TO ACCESS SOME OF HER OWN
TENDENCY TO TURN AWAY. I AM AGREEABLE TO TRYING IT.

There's never an arbitrary *no* from Shannon. There's never a no "on
principle"—there may not, for that matter, be a principle. He's so un-
theoretical, so purely *skilled* that he seems to make decisions and to
practice by the seat of his pants. Nearly literally. What tells him how
long a silence should last? Or how curious a grunt should sound, to
elicit a response?

I once saw a photo of him from many years ago, at the very start
of his practice. He was very thin then, dark-faced, and an ashtray beside him was crammed with cigarette butts. But he already had the

same big chair, his feet already tucked up in it, his face unanxious, intent as if he's listening

—happy—already;
there on the magic carpet
as if he's flying.

9

FIRST HOUR "ON THE COUCH." TALKS ABOUT THE FEELING OF CHANGE IN POSI-
TION—THAT IT IS VERY DIFFERENT, THAT SHE FEELS IN THE WRONG PLACE
(CAN'T SEE PRINTS, PHOTO, ME EXCEPT STOCKING FEET—THAT THERE IS NOTH-
ING TO LOOK AT FOR SOMEONE IN THAT POSITION), THAT SHE IS AWARE OF
DIFFERENT BODILY SENSATIONS (COLD FEET, BACK ON SOFA—ALL SURFACE
SENSATIONS). SHE ASKS IF IT IS OK TO FREE ASSOCIATE AND HOW TO DO IT. I SAY
YES AND SAY IT IS A DIFFICULT SIMPLE THING TO SAY WHATEVER COMES INTO
YOUR MIND. SHE TALKS ABOUT SENSATIONS SOME MORE, THEN TALKS ABOUT
THE DISEMBODIED VOICE FEELING DIFFERENT IN THIS POSITION THAN IN
COMPANY WITH OTHERS, TALKS ABOUT THE VOICE QUALITY OF ONE OF HER STU-
DENTS, THEN MENTIONS NEWS OF HER BROTHER AND HIS WIFE, STEPHEN,
SOMEONE ELSE. I COMMENT THAT THERE SEEM TO SUDDENLY BE A LOT OF PEO-
PLE HERE AFTER HER TALKING ABOUT SENSATIONS FOR A WHILE. SHE SAYS THAT
THAT WAS WHEN SHE FELT SHE WAS FREE ASSOCIATING—THAT THERE ARE A
LOT OF THOUGHTS OF A LOT OF PEOPLE IN HER HEAD.

"ON THE COUCH" SHE CONTINUES ATTENDING TO SENSATIONS. THE UPPER
PART OF HER BODY IS EXPERIENCED DIFFERENTLY FROM THE LOWER AS SHE
HAS HER HANDS ON HER FACE AND STOMACH. AS SHE TALKS HER VOICE GETS

SOFTER AND QUIETER, OFTEN DIFFICULT FOR ME TO UNDERSTAND WHAT SHE IS SAYING. SHE SEEMS TO DRIFT OFF, VERY OCCASIONALLY DOING SOMETHING TO CHECK IF I AM STILL THERE. (I NEED TO MAKE MORE PROMPT NOTES ON THESE SESSIONS AS THE CONTENT IS MUCH LESS OR MUCH DIFFERENTLY STRUCTURED THAN IN THE FACE-TO-FACE INTERACTIONS.)

———————

FANTASY OF WRESTLING WITH ME AND THROWING HER LEGS AROUND ME AND SQUEEZING——PLEASURABLE MIX OF EXERTION, AGGRESSION, PLAY AND EROTICISM. ASKS IF THE FANTASY IS OK. REMARKS HOW UNUSUAL IT IS FOR HER TO ASK A QUESTION THAT MIGHT EVEN REMOTELY GET A NO ANSWER.

———————

FANTASY ABOUT TAKING MY SOCKED FOOT AND MASTURBATING WITH IT. // CRYING MUCH OF YESTERDAY——FEELING LIKE "ALL THE STARCH HAS BEEN WASHED OUT OF ME" // THOUGHTS ABOUT THE TWO FANTASIES ABOUT ME——NO PENETRATION IS IMPORTANT; SOME ASSOCIATION WITH THE CHILDHOOD GAME OF RIDING HORSIE ON FATHER'S KNEE/LEG. // FEELING SKINLESS, SUNK INTO HERSELF, OR ALL ON THE SURFACE LIKE A SOAP BUBBLE, NOT CENTERED——LIKE THE EFFECT HER PARENTS CAN HAVE ON HER——ANXIOUS ABOUT INTERPERSONAL STUFF——LONELY AND IMPINGED UPON——FELT THIS WAY A LOT AS A GIRL. (?) FEELING IS ABOUT EMPTY SPACES, SADNESS, ANXIETY. AFFECTIVE FITS OF ANXIETY, SHAME, BADNESS——ARE THESE DEGENERATIVE TRANSFORMATIONS OF SEXUAL SENSATIONS??

———————

SAYS SHE IS EMBARRASSED AND BEMUSED BY NOT KNOWING WHAT TO DO WITH THE GENITAL FOCUS THAT JUST COMES UP WHEN SHE LETS HERSELF RELAX ON THE COUCH. GOES BACK TO THE TICKLING, LAUGHING AND THE SCENE OF MASTURBATING WITH GIRLFRIENDS. SAYS MOST OF THE SEXUAL PLAY WAS STRUCTURED IN THE S/M NARRATIVE AND FELT QUITE DIFFERENT FROM THE GENITAL

EXCITEMENT SHE WAS DESCRIBING, WHICH SEEMS "OUT OF HAND," LACKING
A NARRATIVE, SHY, FUGITIVE, LIKE MAKING SOMEONE LAUGH.

SCARY DREAM OF BEING ACCUSED OF KILLING SOMEONE WHOM SHE ACTUALLY
HADN'T KILLED. WAS TO BE TAKEN OFF BY THIS MOB AND KILLED AND HER
BODY PUT ON A COMPOST HEAP TO ROT UNTIL THERE WAS NOTHING LEFT BUT
HER HAIR, LONGER THAN SHE HAS IT NOW. // DESCRIBING THE PARANOID
SPACE. SCHEMELESS / UNPROTECTED / PEOPLE MAD AT ME / TOO MUCH GOING
ON TO KEEP TRACK OF / ALL MY FAULT / PUT TO THE TEST BY EVERYTHING /
THINGS I DO HAVING AN EFFECT DISPROPORTIONATE TO MY INTENTION / OTH-
ERS SELF-DESTRUCTING IN WAYS I CANNOT CONTROL (THOUGHT/FANTASY OF
WALKING OUT OF MY OFFICE AND MY WIFE IS THERE, SEVERE AND SAD; E DOES
NOT KNOW IF IT IS SEVERE OR SAD AND DOESN'T HAVE THE INTERPERSONAL
WEAVE TO INQUIRE, NOR TO KNOW IF HER BEING THERE REGISTERS WITH MY
WIFE OR DOESN'T). PROBABLY GOES BACK TO HER MOTHER——PREOCCUPIED,
VIGILANT, DEPRESSED, DRAINED? /// SAYS THAT IF SHE ADMITS TO AWARENESS
SOME KIND OF GENITAL DESIRE WITHOUT A STRUCTURE TO SATISFY IT, IT WILL
BE LIKE WALKING THROUGH THE WORLD WITH A GAPING WOUND. WHY HAVE
DESIRES IF I DON'T KNOW HOW TO SATISFY THEM? // I SAY SHE IS QUITE ADAP-
TIVE AND NOT TOO REACTIVE. REMINDS HER OF STRUCTURE OF HER JEALOUSY:
IT WOULD MAKE HER FRUSTRATED, ANGRY, DESPERATE, BUT JUST AS SOON AS
SHE FOUND A NARRATIVE WAY TO EMPATHIZE WITH HER RIVAL THE ANGER ET
AL. WOULD DISAPPEAR. /// GAPING WOUND, ADOLESCENCE, LOSS OF CLOSED
BODY, OPEN-SECRETING-SMELLY THING, VULNERABLE——NOT ATTRACTIVE, BE-
TRAYAL OF MY MOTHER?

> Lying on the couch
> it's the silences that are
> supposed to spook you
>
> into blurting your
> own, feared Gothic projectiles
> into the long void.

That never happens!
Instead it is as if I'm
inside Shannon's head

when he unspools the
breathless hypothesis that
each second is of

each silence in our
room—giddily welcoming
speculation of

what words may arise
and at what instant they may,
bubbling, between us.

———

REFLECTING ON THE KLEINIAN NOTION OF CHILDREN'S INTERNAL FANTASIES
—I.E., THAT THE WAY KIDS EXPERIENCE SOMETHING LIKE BEING HUNGRY IS
NOT AS A LACK BUT AS SOMETHING INSIDE THEM LIKE A HUNGRY ANIMAL. RES-
ONATES WITH THE AFTERMATH OF DEALING WITH CANCER AND ALL OF THE AL-
TERNATIVE INSIDE BODIES SHE FEELS SHE HAS. SEEMS APT THAT I WOULD
CONTINUE EXPERIENCING MY BODY IN THIS WAY LONG AFTER MOST CHILDREN
WOULD HAVE GIVEN IT UP—THAT I DID NOT HAVE A CLEAR SENSE OF CAUSE
AND EFFECT, OF LESS AND MORE. RELATES TO MY EXPERIENCE OF DIGESTIVE
THINGS, CANCER, HOT FLASHES, SEXUAL THINGS. SHE IS EXPERIENCING A
CHANGE IN HER RELATIONSHIP WITH DEATH—SOMEWHAT THAT IT IS A SIM-
PLE FACT, NOT THAT IT WAITS SOON FOR HER, OR THAT IT IS SOMETHING SHE
SEEKS.

———

"I've noticed a change since we started talking about all this S/M. I
don't seem to be animated by that old fantasy of making you smarter.
This isn't feeling like an exciting experiment now.

"If anything, I'm more struck by the banality of what I'm bringing you—that, and of course the banality of my resistance to it.

"Yeah, I'm a little abashed at the comedown, but

> to tell you the truth
> I feel relieved by it, too,
> the sense of being
>
> a very routine
> patient with one more set of
> none-too-enthralling
>
> erotic triggers
> whom you listen to as you
> listen to others."

———————

DISPLAY AND ANATOMIZATION OF WOMAN'S GENITALS THE FOCUS OF FANTASIES LATE TEENS AND ON——MORE LABIA AND CLITORIS THAN VAGINA——SENSE OF DIS- BELIEF UNDERLIES THOSE FANTASIES, THAT THOSE GENITALS ARE COMICAL OR UNLIKELY AND MYSTERIOUS——INSIDE/OUTSIDE, NEAT/SLOPPY, OPEN/ CLOSED—— EARLIER FANTASIES' MATERIAL WAS OF BACKSIDES, SPANKING, PENISES, CASTRA- TION——ALSO STRUCK WITH HOW UNRELATIONAL THIS IS, UNPEOPLED, AND HOW I DON'T HAVE A "VOCABULARY" FOR SEXUAL RELATIONS BETWEEN PEOPLE.

———————

WHEN SHE TALKS ALOUD TO ME ABOUT THE SEXUAL FANTASIES AND HOW ISO- LATED OR CUT OFF FROM ANY REAL RELATIONSHIPS THEY ARE, THAT MAKES THAT SEPARATION NOT TRUE. BOTHERS ME LOSING ACCESS TO MASTURBATION FANTASY WORLD, BUT NICE TO HAVE THE WARM GLOW OF EROTICISM AROUND DAY TO DAY——NO SENSE OF HOW IT MIGHT BECOME ORGASMIC——WILLING TO EXPERIENCE IT AS AN ADDITION RATHER THAN A LOSS——IT DOES FEEL LIKE ME——PICKING UP ON SENSE OF LACKING A VOCABULARY OR CODES——META- PHOR OF SIGNAL TRANSMITTER/RECEIVER——NOT ADEPT AT TELLING IF I AM

EMITTING A STRONG/WEAK, CLOSE/DISTANT SEXUAL SIGNAL AND HARD TO BE
SURE ABOUT OTHERS' SIGNALS/RECEPTIONS ————IMAGE OF THE SPLAYED,
DISPLAYED, ZONED FEMALE GENITALS—MY RELATION TO GENITAL FEELING IS
SIMILARLY ZONED, ISOLATED—I STRIPPED A LOT OF MEANING AWAY FROM THE
HUMAN BODY WHEN I WAS A KID.

———————

THERE IS A LONG DREAM WHERE E IS MAKING/EDITING A VIDEO OF A DOG
JUMPING DOWN FROM A TABLE. THE SALIENT THING ABOUT THE DOG IS HOW
SMOOTHLY AND SLEEKLY ITS SKIN FITS. THEN E'S MOTHER COMMENTS THAT IT
IS SILLY OF HER TO BE DOING THIS EDITING AS SHE DOESN'T KNOW ANYTHING
ABOUT IT, NOT EVEN ABOUT THE NEED FOR AN ESTABLISHING SHOT. E REALIZES
SHE DOESN'T BUT IS ABLE TO FEEL THAT SHE CAN DO GOOD WORK DESPITE HER
MOTHER'S POINT. —— TO E NOW THIS SUGGESTS A POWERFUL DESCRIPTION OF
HER SITUATION: NO SEXUAL SUBJECT POSITION TO ORGANIZE HER SENSATIONS
AND IMPULSES. SHE WEEPING OVER THIS DESPITE CONFIDENT TONE OF DREAM.
I ALSO COMMENT ON THE AMOUNT OF SKIN AND TEXTURE AND TACTILE CON-
TENTS SHE HAS PRODUCED SINCE GETTING ON THE COUCH. SHE WONDERS IF IT
IS PARTLY A "TYRANNY OF THE VISUAL" THAT OCCURS WHEN ONE'S EYES ARE
OPEN AND CHANGES WHEN SHE LIES THERE WITH HER EYES CLOSED.

———————

"Was I being completely awful last time?"

"Not so I noticed," Shannon answers promptly, "did you feel like
you were?"

"Yeah! Did I ever! Sniveling and whining. Walking out of here, for
some reason all I found myself thinking was, 'Christ, it's a good thing
Shannon doesn't spank.'"

> No doubt he wants to
> cock his brow and ask what makes
> me so sure of *that*,

but instead he sits back, looks blandly interested.

"As a matter of fact . . ." I find myself saying. "There was this dream image that came this morning, just as I was surfacing from sleep . . ."

"?"

"The image was of me, quite cheerfully if not eagerly, pulling down my pants in order to put myself over somebody's lap to be spanked."

"Ah, 'somebody.'"

"Well, you didn't figure corporeally in the dream; but it did feel to be clearly you. Or some relation."

I've told Shannon before about some waking-up dreams like this. There's always some punishment (of me) going on in them. But as my dream state imperceptibly glides toward waking, the consciousness dawns and dawns that it's actually I who am calling the shots—that it's according to my own directions or wishes that the punishment is proceeding.

> Sometimes there's even
> comedy in the dreams: how
> bossy I'm acting!

> It's embarrassing
> other times that no one else
> wants to play this game

> of punishing Eve
> but because it's my dream, they
> have to play along

> and be indulgent—
> and the sense of agency
> as it surfaces

> funkily and with
> such buoyancy from the murk
> of fake compulsion

gives me the great joy
of recognizing my own
pleasure as the law

of the dream. And then
that being so abashed is
also my pleasure—

What's most striking about this, for me, is that such wonder, such cheerful eagerness, such hilarious arias of uncertain agency, never feature in the S/M fantasies of my waking sexuality. Nothing could be more distant! Nothing could be more distant, either, from any way in which I've ever thought the spankings of my childhood to have happened.

Somewhere—the capillaries of my actual pleasure.

———————

DREAM JUST BEFORE WAKING: SHE IS LYING HAVING BEEN COVERED WITH A PLASTER MIXTURE, NAKED, WITH HER LEGS SLIGHTLY SPREAD, AND HAS TO REMAIN MOTIONLESS UNTIL THE PLASTER DRIES. THE SMOOTHNESS OR CRACKING OF THE PLASTER WILL TELL IF SHE HAS MOVED. AS SHE AWAKES, SHE REALIZES THAT THIS IS A FAMILIAR STRUCTURE OF HER SEXUAL FANTASIES AND THAT SOMEHOW SHE IS IN CONTROL OF THE SCENE, EVEN THOUGH THE AGENCY OF THE ACTION IS DISGUISED. REFLECTING, SHE IS AWARE OF THE SEXUAL CONNOTATIONS FOR HER OF THE POSITION OF LYING ON THE COUCH, AND THAT SOMEHOW THESE DREAMS RELATE TO HOW WE HAVE CHANGED THE FORMAT OF OUR THERAPY. I COMMENT THAT SHE IS QUITE ADEPT AT TURNING ANXIETY INTO EXCITEMENT AND ENJOYMENT IN A NUMBER OF SITUATIONS, BUT NOT IN ALL.

———————

JAMES MERRILL DIED YESTERDAY AND E TALKS OF SADNESS AT THAT. READS ME A MERRILL POEM CALLED "THE KIMONO."

. . . Keep talking while I change into
The pattern of a stream
Bordered with rushes white on blue.

———————

HER DIFFUSE GENITALLY CENTERED SENSE OF SEXUALITY HAS RETURNED. SAYS
THAT IT IS HERE AT THE PLACE OF TALKING ABOUT THE EXPERIENCE, THE S/M
FANTASIES, NOT WITHIN THE FANTASIES, THAT THE SENSE OF AN ENJOYING
SUBJECT WITH AGENCY IS POSSIBLE/PERMITTED. WITHIN THE FANTASY IT IS ALL
RESISTANCE AND COMPULSION. [I WONDER IF THIS DESCRIPTION OR SCHEMA
MAY APPLY TO AREAS OTHER THAN JUST SEX.]

"When I look for the most direct pipelines to childhood experience,
here's a big one.

"To begin with: how it feels when I'm with people I think are fond
of me, and who know me well, and who are making gentle fun of me.
I love this sensation. But also feel that I probably love it *too much*, that
it means way too much to me; that this must be visible somehow; and
that the excess of it is liable to make my friends' gentle teasing turn
from laughing with into just plain laughing *at* me.

"Which I hate, being laughed at. It invokes the whole, vicious circle of being 'thin-skinned,' babyish, a sore loser . . . which always only
confirms itself, ratchets up the level of wretched, somatic self-con-
sciousness, making things worse and worse . . .

"There's a particular body sense that goes with this position, too. A
sense that the front of my face is not only engorged with blood, but
somehow almost detachable—detached from me, separate from me,
that I'm living (cowering?) behind it.

"I'm sure there's something in this knife-edge feeling that goes far,
far back."

But Shannon isn't sure he knows the feeling.

"Well," I undertake again, "I could imagine you experiencing it. For
instance if you were doing something with a bunch of other men—

men you liked, but maybe didn't feel too sure of being accepted by—
say you were going out on a boat with a bunch of fishermen, or something, and wanted them to accept you, maybe not to view you as
overeducated and inept—and you managed to say something guyish
or funny that really seemed to bond you with them. Which would
make you feel very safe, and proud. But then as you felt that, you'd also
worry that it might be legible to them how special this bond seemed
to you—and this in itself could turn things around and alienate them.
Like you might laugh too loud or long at your own joke. Isn't that
something you could imagine feeling?"

"Oh, yes. I see now."

Which propels us to the overarching category of feeling: "caught off
balance." "A big one for you," Shannon correctly notes. "A bunch of
things you talk about seem to have this in common."

"Oh, yes," I say, abruptly sitting straight up, planting my feet on the
floor. (Some mix of a formulation suddenly arrived at, and probably
guessing the hour is almost up.) "In fact, I wonder whether it would-
n't be right to say this: what being a grownup means for me is trying
to learn not to be caught off-center in those ways—hardly ever; it's really pretty infrequent for me now.

"But trying to accomplish that somehow

without constructing
a lot of psychic armor.
Cause I really don't

feel I *have* done that . . . ?"
"No. There is no carapace
of psychic armor."

———

FANTASIZES TAKING OFF PANTS—CLOTHED ON TOP AND UNCLOTHED ON BOT-
TOM. (SPANKING RELEVANT? / TOILET TRAINING RELEVANT?) HAVING BOTTOM
EXPOSED A PLUS IN TOILET TRAINING, BUT THEN IN SPANKING IT'S ALL SHAME,
NO PRIDE. THE IDEA THAT THERE WAS A GOOD MIX OF PRIDE SHARED WITH

PARENTS, A BIT OF SHAME, AND A DOSE OF AUTONOMY IN THE TOILET TRAIN-
ING—A PLEASING IMAGE OF HERSELF AS A TODDLER. LATER THE SPANKING HAS
MOSTLY SHAME, WITHOUT PRIDE OR AUTONOMY AND WITH NO AFFECTIVE RE-
LATING BY PARENTS IN THE SPANKING SCENE.

Shannon can't believe I was toilet trained at one! "But back then," I
say, "people *were*." But he says even back then, they weren't; that it's
pretty far out of the line of physiological development. One-year-olds,
he says, don't have the perceptual skills, never mind the muscular
control, to accomplish the task—a complex one that requires feeling
the state of your bowel, knowing when it wants emptying, learning the
ways of a sphincter. "You *can* do it from outside," he says, "plop the kid
on the pot for an hour after every meal. Let them off when they're
done. But that's achieving the end by short-circuiting the process."
    When I ask my mother, it's the usual story.

"Really you toilet
    trained yourself. You couldn't wait
    to be a big girl!"

        To Shannon—then to
    me—this makes so much sense of
    the incoherent

    way that I never
    pieced together a sense of
    my own sexual

    desire, one that would
    have an inner origin
    and radiate out

    making an arc of
    energy that would connect
    a want with an act . . .

SOME REFLECTION ON LATELY DIFFERENT NATURE OF THE THERAPY—E DOES
NOT GO OVER THE HOUR AND WRITE IT UP IN THE WAY SHE USED TO DO, IT
FEELS MORE COLLABORATIVE AND MORE RELAXED TO ME. WE TALK TODAY MORE
SPECULATIVELY ABOUT HER EARLY DEVELOPMENT. SHE WONDERS IF SOME OF
THE FEELINGS ABOUT DEATH AND DEADNESS IN HER HAVE TO DO WITH TOILET
TRAINING, WHICH HER MOTHER FINISHED WITH HER BY AGE 1 AND ONCE
SAID SHE USED A FAIR AMOUNT OF SHAMING TO ACCOMPLISH. E THINKS OF
"ACCIDENTS" AS DISGRACING HERSELF. I WONDER HOW THIS RELATES TO THE
MISCARRIAGE/STILLBIRTH AND HER LEARNING ABOUT DEATH, OR HOWEVER AT
AGE 1 SHE EXPERIENCED HER MOTHER'S BEING PREGNANT AND THEN NOT
HAVING A BABY???

FOCUS SHIFTS TO HER BODY AND AN IMAGE OF A SORT OF GLASS BOTTLE BODY
FILLED WITH A BUBBLY LIQUID, WITH THE BUBBLES CLUSTERING IN DIFFERENT
SPOTS. SHE FEELS THERE CONTINUES TO BE SOME NEW SENSE OF SEXUALITY
WORKING ITS WAY OUT FOR HER, ONE THAT IS NOT AIMED AT ME BUT IS SOME-
HOW IN RELATION TO ME, THAT IS NOT EXACTLY THE SELF-ENCLOSED MASTUR-
BATORY SEXUALITY OF HER PAST. ———RECOUNTS A DREAM OF GOING TO A
DOCTOR IN A SPANISH-SPEAKING COUNTRY TO GET NEW BREASTS, COSMETIC. A
NICE, HANDSOME DOCTOR WITH WHITE GLASSES. WHEN SHE WAKES, SHE WON-
DERS WHAT SHE WANTED THE NEW BREASTS FOR, ANYWAY, AND DOES NOT HAVE
AN ANSWER TO THIS. BRIEFLY ASSOCIATES TO HAVING A SCAR WHERE THE
BREAST WAS REMOVED, HER VALUING OF THE SCAR AS A CLAIM FOR ATTENTION
AND TENDERNESS AND CARE. THAT IF PEOPLE ARE AFRAID *FOR* HER THEY WILL
NOT BE AFRAID *OF* HER.

CONFUSED ABOUT SEX AND WHAT SEXUAL FEELINGS FEEL LIKE—MOVING AND
NOT MOVING, AGENCY AND NOT AGENCY. //RECURRENCE OF HER OLD DREAM OF
FOND CONVERSATION WITH BENJ WHO THIS TIME ASKS WHAT WILL WE DO FOR
MEANING IN OUR LIVES NOW THAT WE HAVE ACHIEVED WHAT WE SET OUT TO

DO IN OUR WORK? SAYS SHE ACTUALLY DOESN'T FEEL LIKE THAT—THAT IT IS
NOT HARD FOR HER TO FIND MOTIVATION AND MEANING. // OTHER DREAMS
LATELY, LONG DISCURSIVE ONES WITH THEMES OF REGRET AND/OR REMORSE.
IN ONE SHE IS LOOKING IN THE MIRROR AND SEES HERSELF REFLECTED AS THE
CHILD IN THE PHOTO FOR THE POETRY BOOK COVER, BUT WITH ONE BREAST
MISSING AND THAT LONG HAIR. TALKS ABOUT THAT BODY AS SLENDER, DIS-
CRETE, RESOLUTE, SELF-CONTAINED. THE GIRL IS JUST BEFORE ALL OF THE TUR-
MOIL OF BECOMING GENDERED COMES DOWN ON HER.

COMES IN WITH SPLITTING HEADACHE WHICH SHE ATTRIBUTES TO THE AFTER-
MATH OF HAVING HOSTED LESBIAN VISITING POET YESTERDAY. SHE NOTES THAT
THE POEMS WERE SEXY, THAT SHE RESONATES WITH MANY OF THE FEELINGS,
BUT "THE THING ABOUT DIRECTING THAT RIGHT TOWARDS ANOTHER PERSON I
JUST DON'T GET." SHE IS STILL THINKING ABOUT LAST SESSION AND THE IMAGE
OF THE KID. SAYS SHE FEELS SPLIT—SEEING HERSELF AS SPOILED VS. SEEING
HERSELF AS VALUABLE. THE SENSE OF SPOILAGE/WASTAGE/RUIN IS PHYSICALLY
AND GENDER-WISE. THE VALUABLE IS PERSONAL, INTELLECTUAL, SPIRITUAL. I
ASK ABOUT THE SPOILED. I'VE RUINED MY BODY OR IT'S RUINED ME. NOTHING
IS GOING TO WORK. I REFUSE OR FAIL GENDER CATEGORIES, NOT IN THE SENSE
OF HOW PEOPLE SEE ME, JUST IN HOW IT IS. (I ASK ABOUT RUINED) NEVER BE
A COMFORTABLE BODY TO INHABIT, NEVER MOVING EASILY, WRONG TEMPERA-
TURE, SPOILED IN TERMS OF NOT BEING INTELLIGIBLY MASCULINE OR FEMI-
NINE (THOUGH TO ME CLEARLY FEMALE). REMEMBERS A POEM HER MOTHER
USED TO RECITE WHICH BEGINS "OH FAT WHITE WOMAN WHOM NOBODY LOVES,
WHY DO YOU WALK THROUGH THE FIELDS IN GLOVES . . . ?" CRYING. ALWAYS
FELT THE POEM WAS POINTED AT HER AND IMPLIED THAT SHE WOULD BE LIKE
THIS, UNLOVED AS SHE MATURED INTO A WOMAN. SHE ISN'T, BUT THE GENDER
AREA IS POISONED AGAINST HER BEFORE SHE EVER GETS A CHANCE TO TRY HER
HAND AT IT.

In New York for the weekend, I'm paused over Merrill's death with a
friend. I've long been haunted by his piece about a trip to Japan, called

"Prose of Departure," in an unfamiliar form: prose interspersed with haiku.

Spangled with haiku is more what it feels like, his very sentences fraying

> into implosions
> of starlike density or
> radiance, then out

into a prose that's never quite not the poetry—

I never really got haiku as a short form. Precious, insipid, I think would have been my words for it. This seems so different. Sweeping into and through the arias, silent impasses, the fat, buttery condensations and inky dribbles of the mind's laden brush.

Josh says it's a seventeenth-century Japanese form called haibun. He's meanwhile been reading Basho's haibun—the form, he says, classically used for narratives of travel.

In the middle of the evening, it comes to me as a possible form for writing of Shannon and me.

A topic that's, of course, long teased with possibility. But the genres I know for undertaking it are so bathetic! If not complaint ("My shrink doesn't understand me. Also he wants me to pay to have sex with him"), then fixation—as our therapy's oddly never fixated—on the truths uncovered, the excavated past.

Or worst, the expert triumphalism of the case history. "And then when I explained . . ."

I've thought about Platonic dialogues—that's getting closer. Or novels, where you needn't know in advance what the subject *is*: a love? A failure? A mess? A bliss?

But that's—prose.

> To notate our strange
> melody, I have some use
> for all the white space.

———————

UP-AND-DOWN WEEKEND——EUPHORIC/UNCENTERED BY HAIKU BOOK PROJ-
ECT——IS IT RELATED TO SEX STUFF? // DREAM——BLEEDING AGAIN WITH THE
DREAM AFFECT MIXED. IS AT A SCHOOL REUNION WITH GIRLS SHE HAS TAUGHT,
AND ALTHOUGH SHE DOES NOT CLEARLY REMEMBER THEM, THEY ARE DEVOTED
TO HER. THEY HAVE GIVEN HER SOMETHING TO WEAR——A SORT OF BABY DOLL
DRESS. SHE THINKS THAT IT WON'T FIT HER BUT IT DOES AND SHE LOOKS GOOD,
TERRIFIC. SHE THINKS, "WHY DON'T I WEAR STUFF LIKE THIS?" WHILE CHANG-
ING SHE NOTICES HER PANTIES AND HER BRA ARE FULL OF BLOOD. SHE HAS
THE SAME REACTIONS——CANCER?, MENSTRUATING AGAIN, SCARED, HOPEFUL,
ETC. EVERYONE LIKES THE DRESS.————TALKING WITH MICHAEL, HE COM-
MENTS THAT HE HAS SOMETIMES FELT THAT HE'S FED HIS "CHILDREN" EVERY-
THING, INCLUDING HIS GENDER.———MORE ABOUT HER SEXUAL FEELINGS
——NAGGING, TOOTHACHE-LIKE RATHER THAN SPECIFICALLY SEXUAL. EVEN AT-
TENDING TO THE FEELING GETS HER INVOLVED IN THE ISSUE OF "SEX
TOWARD . . ."

———————

HAD A THOUGHT ABOUT ME——THAT MAYBE I HAVE SOME IDENTIFICATION
WITH HER LYING THERE ON THE COUCH, TRYING TO HOLD ON TO SEXUAL SEN-
SATIONS AND SPIN A COHERENT THREAD OUT OF THEM. PREVIOUSLY HAD AS-
SUMED I WAS LIKE A STEREOTYPE MALE WITH EASILY ACCESSIBLE AND QUICKLY
ON-AND-OFF SEXUAL FEELINGS.

———————

ON THE COUCH——NO FOCUS, A WASH OF FEELINGS AND THOUGHTS——IS SOME
BACK TO AWARENESS OF THE SEXUAL FEELINGS——IMAGE OF ME PERCHED ON
THE EDGE OF A BIG TEACUP WHICH CONTAINS THE WASH OF FEELINGS AND
THOUGHTS——MIMICKING THE PERCH SHE IS AWARE OF THE PELVIC TENSION
WHICH FEELS SEXUAL——SWITCHES TO IMAGE OF HUMMINGBIRD TASTING/
TESTING THE FLAVOR OF HER SEXUALITY.

———————

DREAM: A NOTEBOOK OF MINE, POEMS, LISTS, DRAWINGS, INCLUDING S/M MA-
TERIAL. A GROUP PUTTING TOGETHER AN AVANT-GARDE SHOW HAS GOTTEN
HOLD OF THE NOTEBOOK, CUT IT UP AND REASSEMBLED IT ALONG WITH ADDED
MATERIALS INTO AN EXHIBIT PIECE, A DIFFERENT OBJECT. INSIDE THE BACK
COVER IS A POCKET WITH LITTLE OBJECTS, FIGURES, STICKERS. MY RESPONSE IS
MIXED——SHOCK AT MY SEXUAL STUFF DISPLAYED, IMPRESSED WITH THE ART
PIECE AS A PIECE——COMPELLING, MAGNETIC, INTERESTING——MY STUFF
LOOKED GOOD, A REAL ACHIEVEMENT, VERY FUNNY.——— OTHER PART OF THE
DREAM: HAL AND I ARE IN JAPAN, EXPLORING. WE NOTICE THAT THEY DON'T
WALK ON THE BARE GROUND BUT ON BOARDWALKS OF THIN BOARDS OR REEDS.
IT IS NOT STURDY ENOUGH FOR ME——SIZE, WEIGHT——AND IT BOUNCES, BUCK-
LES BUT DOES NOT BREAK. THEN IT BEGINS TO FEEL LIKE A TRAMPOLINE——I LAY
BACK, ENJOY IT, BOUNCE UP AND DOWN——NICE FEELING TO LIE HERE, ENJOY
IT, NOT TO TRY TO GET ANYWHERE.

I SAID THAT I DIDN'T FIND ANYTHING VERY INTERESTING IN THE DREAMS
AND E ASKS WHY. AS I TALK IT IS CLEAR THAT THE COMMENT COMES SOME
FROM MY CONFUSION AND PREOCCUPATION WITH THE ARM PAIN I'M HAVING,
SOME FROM THE FACT THAT THE DREAM WOULD HAVE LED US TO TALK ABOUT
HER AND ME AND I WAS TRYING TO AVOID TALKING ABOUT ME AND MY SLIPPED
DISK, AND MORE TO THE POINT, I EXPERIENCED HER LYING ON THE COUCH
AWAY FROM ME AS AN ABANDONMENT WHILE I WAS IN PAIN AND WAS ANGRY
ABOUT THAT.

AS WE TALK THE PAIN IS GONE.

———————

STOPPED MASTURBATING——NOT THAT I DON'T FEEL SEXY——CONSTANT SEXUAL
ENERGY WANTING TO TURN INTO MOVEMENT, AFFECTION, WRITING, EVERY-
THING. // STILL A FAIR AMOUNT OF FREE-FLOATING ANXIETY AND SADNESS——A
CONVERSATION IS GOING ON THAT I DON'T KNOW MUCH ABOUT THE CONTENT
OF YET. GROIN LEVEL——WARM SEXUAL ENERGY; LUNG LEVEL——ANXIETY; EYE
LEVEL——SADNESS. TENSION IN SHOULDERS AND NECK, KINESTHETIC CON-

———————

I see that one of the main ways I'm using Shannon is as an excuse to be more withdrawn.

All those conversations where my friends here ask what goes on in therapy that's so absorbing . . . and

I say, over and
over, "Well, it's just—oh, it's
just—*interesting.*"

It reminds me of all the unsuccessful job interviews, in the years before I got professionalized, when I'd be asked to describe my dissertation and

gazing off into
outer space, would murmur, "Oh,
it's . . . complicated."

It's hard to say why the return to this unskilled, unsociable demeanor feels just right.

It's as though there were something true, or vital, in all that old shyness. A thread for the labyrinth.

———————

TANT. SORRY." (THIS WAY THEY LET HER AVOID THE TIRINGNESS OF JUST BEING
IN HER OWN LIFE.)

———————

POETRY BOOK!!! SHE WAS IN NY OVER THE WEEKEND AND CELEBRATED THE
BOOK'S BEING OUT. WHEN SHE GETS BACK SHE GETS CALL FROM HAL ABOUT
THEIR DOCTOR IN NY WHO TURNS OUT TO HAVE AN AIDS RELATED INFECTION.
SHE AND HAL ARE STUNNED. EDITING GARY. SHE FEELS SOMEHOW THAT HER
PRESENT WAY OF MOVING BETWEEN THE LIVING AND THE DEAD IS OBSCENE,
DIRTY (DIRT AS MATTER OUT OF PLACE). TOO, THE KNOWLEDGE THAT HER DOC-
TOR IS ILL FEELS LIKE IT CUTS HER OFF FROM BEING ABLE TO DIE. SHE EXPERI-
ENCES HER FIRST TASTE OF BEING AFRAID OF DEATH.

Still immersed, morning till night, in Gary's book. The archaic
fragrance of profanation around the project only gets more insistent.
A surprise.

I always seemed to feel I could turn back and walk through the
flames, protected by the purity of my heart.

I think I thought that an unswerving immersion could make the
task feel daily rather than uncanny.

> It turns out to be
> easy and natural for
> something to be both.

———————

TALKS ABOUT HER CURRENT DRIVE TO DOCUMENT HERSELF AND OTHERS AS
HAVING SOME RELATIONSHIP TO AN AWARENESS OF DEATH, THAT SHE WANTS TO
LEAVE A SENSE OF HER RELATIONALITY, AFFECTION AND FRIENDS. SHE NOTES A
SENSE IN HER THAT BEING AND DOING ARE QUITE OVERLAPPING AND SOME-
WHAT INDISTINGUISHABLE.

CAN SHE SEE MY NOTES FOR HAIKU BOOK? // FREE-FLOATING CREATIVITY LATELY. SUDDENLY LOTS OF ARTS AND CRAFTS FASCINATION.

Where have they come from, the luscious materials that have suddenly been wooing, feeding my fingers with such solicitous immediacy? And how long has this been going on?

Sure, I used to sew my own clothes, incompetently—back when I had time and no money instead of the opposite. The phrase "arts and crafts" has long made me drool at auctions, as it used to at Girl Scout camp.

But this is so different! And so out of the blue that Shannon and I joke there must be a new tumor pressing on the Sculpey node in my brain. Polymer clay in every color, and paint, and silk kimono scraps— I've started to elope from my school and writing, flying toward this stuff with the stealth, joy, almost the guilt of adultery.

It's strange, because I'm excited about writing—at least the one project, Shannon's. But this thrills me (I don't think I've had quite this feeling before) because it is so *not* writing.

Writing, my perfectionism gets all over everything. I wrestle and contort to keep it at bay long enough for words to get onto the screen. Like Michelangelo knowing what's supposed to emerge from the marble block, my task is to excise everything that isn't *that*. Maybe it's called "knowing what you're doing"; it feels less and less good.

But in this other, indiscriminate realm, that conscience has no foothold. What am I doing? Messing with "stuff." Having materials in my hands; seeing, at an instant of pause and speculation, whether there's something satisfying, something surprising to me, that they *almost* are.

> Little to ask! When
> they turn into anything
> (lovely)—I'm in joy.

———————

WED. NIGHT WAS NO SLEEP, +++ ANXIETY ABOUT GETTING MY NOTES AND HOW SADISTIC SHE CAN BE IN READING SOMEONE ELSE'S WRITING——AFRAID SHE WILL KILL ME, SPOIL ME AS A SOURCE OF NURTURANCE FOR HER WITH SADISM ABOUT HOW I WRITE. HER MOTHER THE ENGLISH TEACHER. IF SHE KILLS ME FOR HERSELF SHE WILL BE KILLING HERSELF. BUT IN THE MORNING SHE RE-CALLS HOW RESILIENT HER SENSE OF ME FOR HER HAS BEEN SO FAR. I GIVE HER MY NOTES.

———————

DIFFICULTY LATELY IN INVOKING ME AS SAFE, COMFORTING——WONDERING IF THE WRITING PROJECT HAD DESTROYED THAT ABILITY, BLAMING SELF FOR GREEDINESS? // POSSIBILITY OF BLEACHING HAIR (STEPHEN'S IDEA)——RELATES TO EXPERIENCING BODY DIFFERENTLY ESPECIALLY SEXUALLY. // PRIDE MARCH TOPLESS WOMEN WITH TWO BREASTS——ENVY. // DREAM——STEALING STUFF FROM PARENTS FOR A BOOK BUT CAN'T FIND CAR SHE'S HIDDEN IT IN——IMPOUNDED BY POLICE——ANXIETY. //

———————

I WAS SO AFRAID OF MY FATHER, AND AM NOT ANYMORE, SO I DON'T KNOW HOW TO GET TO THINKING ABOUT IT (WHAT BROUGHT THIS UP?)——SOME-THING TO DO WITH ANGER ———ALSO WITH READING YOUR NOTES AND SEE-ING YOU AS A REASSURING VERSION OF HIM——THE NOTES ARE TOLD MOSTLY FROM MY POINT OF VIEW, AND LIKE FATHER SOMEHOW——ACCEPTING, SWEET——BUT THE ANGER——

———————

It's hard for me to admit to Shannon, around this time, a habit I have on gray days or early evenings, when I'm sad or ragged, of driving past the corner of Ninth and Main streets, casting my eyes for solace up four stories to the lit-up

honeyed cell of his
availability to
someone—if not me.

————

AGAIN ON MISSING ME WHILE IN NYC AND HOW SOON SHE SLIPPED BACK INTO
A NEUROTIC STANCE OF COPING WITH THINGS. THE WRITING PROJECT——THE
EDGE BETWEEN "WRITING AS" ORDINARY AND EXTRAORDINARY——UNABLE LAST
WEEK TO FEEL IN TOUCH WITH HERSELF AS ORDINARY. //WONDERING: MANIC
SPELL? NOT IN A CLASSIC SENSE ANYWAY. // DREAM——A BEAUTIFUL ONE OF A
BUILDING THAT IS A UNIVERSITY CUM MUSEUM CUM LIBRARY. WHEN YOU GET
ONTO A FLOOR, BESIDES BOOKS THERE ARE WHOLE LANDSCAPES OF THE TOPIC
AREA THAT YOU CAN EXPLORE. THE ONLY ANXIETY IN THE DREAM IS MINOR,
NOT BEING SURE WHERE HER HOME FLOOR IS.

————

I ASK ABOUT HOW IT IS TO BE WEARING SKIRTS——E SAYS ENJOYING. // DREAM
ABOUT GARY——NOT UPSET, JUST HAPPY TO HEAR HIS VOICE. // FEELING SEXY,
DIRECTLY RELATED TO BEING AWARE OF WEARING SHORT SKIRTS. LITTLE GIRLS
IN SHORT SKIRTS, SHOWING OFF THEIR PANTIES——KNOWN SOME ADULTS WHO
DO. HOW MUCH DELIGHT I GET OUT OF JUST BEING SILLY. / SHORT SKIRTS——
TICKLING——SEXUAL SENSATIONS——VIOLENCE——OUIJA BOARD (FOCUS DISSI-
PATES) WHAT DO YOU THINK? (SUGGEST SHE STAY WITH THE SEXUAL FEELINGS
AND THOUGHTS) SENSATIONS——TYLER TALKING ABOUT LOCKER ROOMS AS A
KID, THE FANTASY OF A LINE OF BOYS BEING SPANKED BY GYM COACH——WARM
SPACE OF ATTENTION AND LOVE——NOTES CONSTRICTION IN CHEST, LOSING
TOUCH WITH LOWER BODY——HARD TO THINK/TALK ABOUT. REFOCUS——FEEL-
ING STRONGLY "WHAT DO I WANT WITH THIS?!, WHAT DO I DO WITH THIS?!
WHAT WOULD BE THE POINT."—— ORANGE-YELLOW ENERGY LIKE ORANGE JUICE
GOING THROUGH ME, SENDING ME SINGING OUT INTO THE WORLD——THEN
WHY THIS ONE COLOR, WHY JUST THIS ENERGY CULTIVATED ——OTHER REDDER
ENERGY, DEEPER, MORE GRAVITY, FEELS VERY DIFFERENT——MAGIC CARPET TRY-

ING TO LIFT ME UP——FIRST TIME I'VE EVOKED THAT HERE, THAT FEELING IN
WHICH SO MUCH HAS LIVED FOR ME.

—————

DISCOURAGED AND HOPELESS, AND AT THE EDGE OF STUFF WITH ME—ME IN
(SHE SURMISES) A PATERNAL SEDUCTIVE MODE HAVING ASKED HOW IT FELT TO
WEAR SHORT SKIRTS. THAT RIVETS MY ATTENTION, EXCITES AND INTERESTS ME,
BUT ALSO DISTURBS ME—POSSIBLY SOME KIND OF ADOLESCENT DYNAMIC,
LOOMING CONSEQUENCES BUT NO SPECIFICS—I FEAR EVERYTHING—WANT-
ING SEX WITH YOU AND YOUR BEING UNINTERESTED OR POLITELY BUT HUMILI-
ATINGLY REFUSING—YOUR WANTING SEX WITH ME OR BEING AROUSED BY MY
AUTOEROTICISM, THIS BEING DISRUPTIVE, HIJACKING MY FEELINGS/NEEDS/
AGENDA BECAUSE YOU ARE IMPORTANT TO ME. AND WHAT AM I DOING ENGAG-
ING THIS QUESTION OF SEX BETWEEN PATIENT AND THERAPIST ANYHOW? IS IT
MY QUESTION? POSSIBILITIES AND THREATS DISRUPT MY RELATIONSHIP TO MY
DESIRES IN EARLY ADOLESCENCE—THE VITAL PHYSICALITY I HAVE WITH
MICHAEL, STEPHEN EXTENDS IN HERE TOO. // — SUSPENDED STATE HEDGED
AROUND WITH FEARS, ALL OF WHICH ARE CONTRADICTORY AND NONE OF
WHICH CAN BE FOUND TO BE A "BOTTOM-LINE FEAR"—ELABORATES—(WHY SO
ANXIOUS?) WITH WOMEN I AM IMMOBILIZED—NOT IMMOBILIZED WITH YOU,
MORE SPACE FOR PLAY WITH YOU THAN WITH WOMEN. IT IS SUCH A PLAUSIBLE
STORY—GIRL WHO HAS NOT GOTTEN LOVE TO ENTIRELY TRUST FROM MOTHER,
HAVING INTENSE INTIMACIES WITH MEN IN A MATERNAL GUISE, AND THAT
STRUCTURE THREATENED BY A HETEROSEXUAL OVERLAY OR IMPOSITION. (I SAY
NEEDS MORE SALT AS A STORY—DOESN'T CATCH SOMETHING OF THE ANXIETY
OR THE ANGER OR . . . ?)

(TWO THINGS FROM ME—WAKING THINKING RE SEXUAL INTEREST IN E,
A PHRASE THAT I THINK COMES FROM ADOLESCENCE OR JUST A BIT LATER—
I WOULD IF I COULD BUT I CAN'T SO I WON'T; AND THINKING THAT IT IS NO-
TABLE THAT WE ARE BACK TO THE POINT OF MY NOT BEING GAY BEING SOME-
THING OF A PROBLEM POTENTIALLY—OR IS IT AN OPPORTUNITY.)

—————

SHE FEELS THAT ONE OF THE THINGS SHE HAS GOTTEN IN THERAPY IS A MORE
REALISTIC SENSE AND UNDERSTANDING OF HER POWER. SHE FEELS LESS AND LESS
THAT POWER (INTELLECTUAL, SPIRITUAL, ARTISTIC, ETC.) IS EITHER BOUNDLESS
OR NOTHING, EITHER THE OVERBLOWN BALLOON OR THE SUDDENLY DEFLATED
BALLOON. "MORE LIKE A SLEEPING BAG WITH MANY SEPARATE AIR COMPART-
MENTS—A SINGLE PUNCTURE WON'T FLATTEN IT." RELATES THIS TO EMPHASIS
ON TALENTS RATHER THAN GENIUS. ALSO RELATED TO HANDICRAFT PASSION?
BIG PLEASURES W/OUT BIG GOALS. WITH THIS HAS COME A POSSIBLE SENSE OF
AGENCY THAT MAY NOT LIE ONLY IN EXTREMES OF GRANDIOSITY OR ABJECTION.
BUT SHE RETURNS TO THE QUICKNESS OF HERSELF TO FEEL "I SHOULDN'T BE
GIVEN THIS"— "IT'S NOT GOOD FOR ME." WONDERS IF THIS IS SOME SENSE OF
HAVING BEEN GIVEN BAD FOOD SOMETIME EARLY. IT RELATES TO THE FACT
OF ALL THE WRONG WAYS OF ASKING FOR THINGS THAT THERE WERE IN HER
FAMILY.

———

MOTHER'S VISIT THIS WEEKEND—TALK TO HER ABOUT INCLUDING RELATION-
SHIP WITH W. IN BOOK. OKAY WITH HER. E PROUD! IDEA THAT THE PARENTAL
MONOLITH MADE ANY OEDIPAL NEGOTIATIONS IMPOSSIBLE—E AND NINA AS
KIDS ALWAYS THOUGHT, "YOU TWO HAD NO BUSINESS HAVING KIDS; YOU ONLY
HAVE EYES FOR EACH OTHER"—YOUR ANXIOUS CLINGING TO THE IMAGE OF
NUCLEAR FAMILY CURTAILED SO MANY POSSIBILITIES FOR YOU—ETC. SOME-
HOW WANT YOU (RITA) TO HAVE BEEN BRAVER, MORE FOCUSED, MORE SERIOUS
ABOUT WHAT YOU THOUGHT AND WANTED, AND ABOUT YOUR DESIRES. IF I'M
ASKED WHERE AM I IN ALL THIS, I DON'T KNOW; CAN'T TELL ON WHOSE BEHALF
I FEEL THIS INJURY.

———

DEATH OF ONE OF EVE'S FINCHES PROMPTS MOTHER TO TALK ABOUT NINA'S
PARAKEET FROM CHILDHOOD AND RITA'S LETTING IT OUT BECAUSE SHE FELT
ANIMALS SHOULD BE FREE—AND ITS GETTING EATEN BY THE CAT—HA, HA!
TRUE?? THROUGH THE DAY MOTHER TALKING IN THAT FAKEY EMOTIONAL WAY
ABOUT HOW BAD SHE FELT, AND E MUST HAVE FELT, ABOUT THE FINCH. BUT

E IS REALLY VERY UNSETTLED BY THE BIRD'S DEATH. R CAN CARICATURE AN
EMOTION IN SUCH A WAY THAT YOU THEN CAN'T FEEL/HAVE EMOTIONS? RE-
LATES TO WHY I THOUGHT THREE YEARS AGO THAT I DIDN'T HAVE ANY EMO-
TIONS—VERY HARD AS A CHILD TO HAVE EMOTIONS, A SENSE OF THEIR CLAIMS
OR WEIGHT, REALITY, WHEN EMOTIONAL FIELD IS PREEMPTIVELY DISCREDITED
IN THIS FASHION—CAN SEE IT IN NINA, THE DENIAL OF EMOTIONS, ESPE-
CIALLY ONES ABOUT COMPASSION, THEN WHEN SHE DOES RECOGNIZE AN EMO-
TION, HOW INFLEXIBLE SHE HAS TO BE IN ORDER TO BE SURE OF HOLDING ON
TO IT AS HERS. THIS RELATES TO WHY A DEPRESSION OR SADNESS, SO IN-
TRACTABLE, SEEMED A GUARANTEE OF MY REALITY—THE DEFENSE OF "THAT'S
JUST HOW SHE IS."

———

DREAM WITH HAL AND ME AND MY MOTHER. HAL AND I HAVING SEX IN A BIG
OLD HOTEL—ENJOYING—BUT I HAVE TO FIND MY MOTHER—LOOKING FOR
HER—REALIZE THAT I FORGOT TO NOTICE WHETHER EITHER OF US HAD AN
ORGASM—DISCONCERTING.——HOTEL UNDER RENOVATION AND THERE ARE
EXPOSED FLOORS, WHOLE SIDES OPEN WITH NO WALLS. CANNOT GET TO THE
DINING ROOM THAT MY MOTHER IS IN FROM WHERE I AM: ORIGINALLY TWO
DIFFERENT BUILDINGS WITH DIFFERENT FOUNDATIONS. THEN THERE TURNS
OUT TO BE A WAY—IF YOU GO AROUND AND THROUGH A BACK ENTRANCE.—
—THE DREAM LEAVES E DELIGHTED WITH THIS PORTRAYAL OF HER SEXUALITY
AT THIS TIME—THE EXPOSED STRUCTURE, INCOHERENCE OF LEVELS, THE CON-
FUSION OF HAL AND HER MOTHER; QUESTION OF ORGASM JUST FLOATING OUT
THERE.

10

HAIKU AND CRAFTS YES

I'm embarrassed—not enough to stop—at the hours and hours I waste with Shannon trying to account for the crafts mania; but more and worse, trying to believe I'm even allowed this vast pleasure. Who knew the old superego had so much blood in her?

It does seem quite a strangeness—the floating downstream with a current that's so resolutely wordless. As though in all its modesty, its refusal to generate propositions, selves, ideas, this might be a cataclysmic change disguised as an unassuming indulgence. As though if I let my

> habitual *yes*
> stretch this far there could never
> be another no.

––––––––

NECK PAIN!! / TEARFUL, FEELING BAD. WILL CONTACT M.D. TODAY.

––––––––

SILK WORK—TURNING FABRIC INTO OTHER FABRIC / CHILDHOOD BLANKET WITH THE SATIN BINDING / SKIN HUNGER / THE FASCINATION EVERYONE HAD WITH HOW SILKY MY SKIN WAS / BRO'S PILLOW PIFFO, HIS DROOLING, "MAKING FISHES" ON IT / MAY SAY SOMETHING ABOUT HOW HUNGRY OUR SKIN WAS FOR TOUCH, BUT ALSO ABOUT OUR HAVING THE PERMISSION TO DEVELOP AUTONOMOUS RESOURCES/ THE DOWNSIDE OF BEING SILKY WAS THAT SOMEHOW I WAS AN OBJECT FOR OTHERS TO SATISFY THEIR TOUCH NEEDS, NOT MINE / TREASURE SCRAPS OF SILK / SOMEHOW THE SILK AND SHIT GO TOGETHER—THE WASTE PRODUCTS, FANTASIES OF SELF-SUFFICIENCY, NOT DEPENDENT, SPINNING STRAW INTO GOLD.

———

THE MASSAGE—STIFF NECK FOR A COUPLE MONTHS—MAYBE FROM THE COUCH, OR THE STRESS FROM CRAFT ACTIVITIES—MY BUM SHOULDER. DREAM THAT SHE WAS TO BUY 12 SCREENS TO HIDE THE DOORS THAT LED TO SPACES UNDER THE EAVES IN THE ATTIC (HER PARENTS' HOUSE) IN WHICH SHE WAS LIVING. SHE HAD LITTLE MOTIVATION FOR DOING THIS BUT HAD PICKED OUT 6 OF THE SCREENS. HAVING A TALK IN THE DREAM WITH EITHER HER MOTHER OR FATHER AND BEING UNUSUALLY CANDID WITH HER/HIM ABOUT HER LACK OF MOTIVATION AND HER FEELING DEPRESSED. FELT SHE WAS BEING UNDERSTOOD. SCENE SHIFTS TO THE BEACH WHERE SHE IS ARRANGING PIECES OF TRANSLUCENT COLORED GLASS IN THE COLORS OF THE SAND, SEA AND SKY. SHE LOOKS BEHIND HER AND SEES THAT A HUGE WAVE IS COMING, BEARING DOWN ON HER, TOO LATE TO RUN, LETS IT ENGULF HER, REALIZES IT IS ACTUALLY NOT SO TERRIFYING.

———

GOOD WORK ON AN ATTRACTIVE WOVEN SCARF, THE PRODUCT OF THE WEEKEND'S LEARNING HOW TO WORK WITH THE TABLE LOOM. TACTILE, NONVERBAL, REGRESSIVE, ENJOYABLE. LACKING THE CONSTANT ALERTNESS IN HER WRITING ABOUT BEING OR BECOMING THE RIGHT PERSON TO DO IT. // TWICE E IS IN THE

MIDDLE OF PARSING THE THREADS OF INFLUENCES AND MEANINGS OF SOME
PART OF THIS OR SOME TOPIC AND THE THREAD OF THE REASONING GETS
LOST——NOT SURE WHAT THIS IS, MORE THAN JUST BEING PREOCCUPIED WITH
WEAVING . . .

———

RESISTANCE TO GOING BACK TO THE *DIALOGUE ON LOVE* IS THAT PRODUCTION
OF THE FIRST PERSON IS BOTH LABOR INTENSIVE AND FELT TO BE CONSTRAIN-
ING, THAT THERE WERE EMOTIONAL REGISTERS THAT WEREN'T AVAILABLE
WHILE GENERATING FIRST PERSON. A TEXTURE BOOK WOULDN'T NEED TO HAVE
A FIRST PERSON AT ALL, ANY MORE THAN WEAVING ITSELF DOES. THAT RHYMES
WITH A LOT OF STUFF FOR ME——THE BUDDHIST STUFF, MANIA FOR MAKING
UNSPEAKING OBJECTS, THE CHILDHOOD EXPERIENCE OF TRAVELING IN THE
CAR WITH THE FAMILY IN THE DARK . . . EVEN FANTASY OF "SILVERY VOICE."

> The cars, each of us,
> bubbles of the same dark, strung
> in a dark necklace.

———

I can't remember if it's Michael or Stephen who first shows me Sogyal
Rinpoche's *Tibetan Book of Living and Dying*. Of course I head straight
for the chapters on how to die, which feel awfully alien; but as I start
to read from the beginning, something else happens.

One assumption I realize, with surprise, I've seen before in
Proust: that when

> the truth comes to you,
> you recognize it because
> it makes you *happy*.

———

FINAL FINCH (OF THE 3 STEPHEN GAVE HER) DIES, AND E DREAMS OF A LINE
OF DEAD BIRDS IN BASEMENT WITH UNDERGROUND PIPES OF POISON GAS AND
SOME MACHINERY WHICH BRINGS THEM THERE TO BE KILLED. E'S SENSE THAT
WHILE SHE MAY NURTURE ADULTS IN HER MAGICAL THINKING MANNER, THE
NURTURING OF SMALLER LIVING THINGS IS SOMETHING SHE IS NOT ABLE TO
DO. HER OLD DREAMS, E.G., OF HAVING A CHILD AND FORGETTING TO FEED IT
AND BEING REMINDED OF THAT BY FINDING IT DEAD. RELATED TO THE LONG
HELD SENSE THAT IF I LOOK AWAY FROM SOMEONE I AM AFRAID TO LOOK BACK
BECAUSE THEY MIGHT BE DEAD, NOT CONTINUOUSLY ANIMATED BY MY GAZE.

———

Raveled mother for
whom three might as easily
have been 300—

———

HAVING BONE SCAN FOR NECK PAIN FRI. TALKED WITH MOTHER WHO MEN-
TIONS IN PASSING THAT SHE HAD "THINGY" REMOVED FROM HER LEG, BUT IT
WASN'T HEALING, BUT SHE DIDN'T WANT TO GO BACK TO THE DOCTOR. WHEN
E ASKS WHAT KIND OF THINGY, SKIN CANCER? MOTHER SAYS YES, BUT WHEN E
ASKS IF MELANOMA, MOTHER SAYS YES, NO, DO NOT KNOW, DOES IT MAKE A DIF-
FERENCE? (THIS FROM R., WHO TOOK CARE OF SON-IN-LAW DYING WITH
MELANOMA.) WHEN E SAYS THAT MELANOMA IS THE FAST-GROWING KIND,
MOTHER SAYS WELL I'M A SLOW PERSON SO IT PROBABLY WAS A SLOW-GROWING
KIND OF CANCER. E CAN SEE HER OWN SOMETIMES GAY AVOIDANCE OF COM-
PLAINT, BUT MORE, SHE UNDERSTANDS BETTER THE ORIGIN OF ANXIETY SHE
FEELS IN STUBBORNLY NEEDING TO FIND OUT AND INSIST ON FACTUAL INFOR-
MATION ESPECIALLY WHEN GRIM. THE OTHER IDEA IS THAT E LETS HERSELF
FANTASIZE FURTHER ABOUT WHAT MIGHT BE WRONG WITH HER AS A WAY OF
GETTING ACCESS TO MORE KLEINIAN/CHILDHOOD THINKING/FANTASIZING
ABOUT THINGS INSIDE HER BODY.

HAD SCAN OF NECK FRI. TO RULE OUT ANYTHING MORE THAN MUSCLE STRAIN
AS CAUSE OF THE NECK PAIN——TURNS UP A SPINAL METASTASIS OF THE BREAST
CANCER OF ALMOST 6 YEARS AGO. I ASK WHAT IT MEANS. SAYS IT MEANS SHE
WILL DIE OF THIS——NOT NECESSARILY SOON THOUGH, AS CANCER SEEMS AN IN-
DOLENT ONE AND SO FAR ONLY IN E'S BONES. 2 YRS–5 YRS? SOME LIVE A
DECADE OR MORE. REACTION SO FAR IS A LITTLE RELIEF OF THE "OTHER SHOE"
VARIETY AND JUST DEALING WITH THE HUGE LOGISTICS OF MORE WORKUPS,
NECK BRACE, PLANS FOR RADIATION THERAPY, WHAT TO DO ABOUT THE SEMES-
TER'S TEACHING, ETC. IN SOME SENSE THIS STILL A REACTION TO THE CANCER,
WITH HER REACTION AS IT RELATES TO HER LIFE STILL TO REGISTER.

> Phones just outside the
> clinic door.
> > Impermanence
> arrives so quickly!

TWO DREAMS——MEDICAL CHECKUP IN BUILDING MADE OVER FROM ROMAN-
ESQUE CATHEDRAL——E ARRIVES WITH HAL, THEN IS WITH TWO NURSES AND
NOTICES SHE IS SEPARATED FROM HAL, CONCERNED THAT HE WILL BE WORRIED
AND UNABLE TO FIND THEM——EXAM BY HER ONCOLOGIST AND AN OLDER M.D.,
HER ONCOLOGIST HAS CANCER NOW AND THE OLDER M.D. HAS HAD IT, HAS
SHIRT OFF AND SCARS ON HIS TORSO. MOVING AROUND IN THE BUILDING E
CATCHES GLIMPSE OF A HIGH, ROUND-ARCHED ATTIC ROOM SOMEONE HAS JUST
LEFT, EMPTY NOW BUT FULL OF GOLDEN YELLOW LIGHT FOR READING, AND
FEELS A LONGING TO BE THERE——RESULT OF TESTS IS BENIGN, THOUGH, AND
SHE IS SORROWFUL WITH SOME OF THE "DO I BELONG IN THIS FAMILY?" FEEL-
ING // SECOND DREAM OF STAGE OR GYM WITH PEOPLE DANCING——SHE IS SUP-
POSED TO GO UP TO SOMEONE AND TAKE A COAT OR SHAWL THEY ARE WEARING
——SEES POOPIE, HER MOTHER'S FATHER, AND TAKES HIS SHAWL GENTLY. //
POOPIE WAS THE LEAST FORMALLY EDUCATED, LOOKED AT THE EVENTS OF LIFE
IN A BEMUSED WAY, SWEET, RECESSIVE, A LITTLE LIKE HAL——GUILT ABOUT HIM

AND NANNY AS THEY WERE SICK AND DIED WHILE E WAS SO DEPRESSED AND
SHE DID NOT VISIT WHEN SHE MIGHT HAVE.

I tell Shannon—like
he couldn't guess—that Buddhism's
conscious love of

rest, death, nonbeing,
are more congenial to
me than the Western

heroic thrust for
individuation and
survival (which seems

plain phony to me).
    I like the explanation
Robert Thurman gives

in his introduction to *The Tibetan Book of the Dead.* "When we see this
equation [the Enlightenment one between death and oblivion] we can
understand at once why materialists scoff at spiritual or religious
forms of liberation. Why would they need it? They have already guaranteed themselves permanent rest. They have a guaranteed nothingness waiting for them, obtained without the slightest effort on their
part, without ethical sacrifice, without realization, without developing
any skill or knowledge. All they have to do is fall asleep, a skill they
have already cultivated during thousands of nights.

"But what is it that provides them the guarantee of a restful nothing awaiting them after death? . . . The answer is, obviously, that they
have no grounds at all for this belief. It is merely a belief based on
brave assertion, corroborated by many other believers, all without a
shred of evidence, reinforced by constant repetition and dogmatic in-

sistence. It provides ultimate comfort, satisfying their religious urge to have a complete sense of reality. This comfortingness might give rise to suspicion or doubt, so is disguised for the materialist by the pretense that nothingness is something frightening, something undesirable, a bitter pill that he or she, the brave modern human grown-up, has learned to swallow."

———

DREAM WITH HER IN SESSION AND MY SAYING INSTEAD OF TALKING I WOULD PLAY THE PIANO, A PIECE WRITTEN FOR THE CROWN AND BEING SENT TO THE UNREBELLIOUS DISSIDENTS IN THE NORTH. SHE FINDS THE PIECE RELAXING AND THE CONCEPT OF MUSIC BEING SENT TO THE UNREBELLIOUS DISSIDENTS TO ENFOLD THEM INTO THE SPHERE OF THE CROWN FASCINATING.

———

Humiliating to me, but when mortality gets personal—so suddenly—the thought of hell refuses to go away. I'm a good rationalist, but it hovers around, and a couple of bad nights give me a crash course in how it can colonize, infect the thought of dying.

Worse, though, it just won't make sense to me, hell. It has nothing to do with my belief. There are five of the Ten Commandments, say, that engage my actual sense of the right and the wrong; and to put it mildly, the people and institutions that are insistent about hell engage it a lot less. Could I really suffer eternally for breaking sanctions that can only seem to me like wicked gibberish?

You'd think my heart could dismiss the possibility of a universe so arbitrary

and at the same time
so punitive . . .

                    "But wait till
your father gets home."

That we each die alone and must work out our salvation in our own way—these seem most urgent spurs, no longer truisms at my new juncture.

———————

EVENTS AT DINNER WITH MIKE AND JON——CHOKING, ALMOST THROWING UP ——THIS IS WHAT IT IS TO BE SICK. (WORSENING SORE THROAT SECONDARY TO THE RADIATION.)——SOMETHING OF A NARCISSISTIC BLOW AND DISTURBINGLY FRIGHTENING TO OTHERS. FEELS A NEED NOT TO BE MESSY ABOUT EVEN BEING THIS SICK. ALSO THE OUTER-SPACE-LOOKING NECK BRACE——NOT BOTHERED AT ALL ABOUT LOOKING WEIRD——UNCHARACTERISTIC INDIFFERENCE TO STIGMA.

———————

GLOOMY——MAKING A WILL, AWARE OF THE PEOPLE SHE HAS TAKEN UNDER HER CARE, PROTECTION AND NURTURANCE WHOM SHE IS NOW LEAVING. SHE AND THEY MUST LEARN SHE IS NOT INDISPENSABLE. BUT ALSO, SOME MOOD OF ELATED, RUTHLESS SELF-INDULGENCE——GIDDILY LIKING NOT TO WORK, NOT TAKING RESPONSIBILITY FOR OTHERS. THE ABSENCE OF ANY AGENCY FOR HER IN THE CANCER MAKES IT EASIER TO SHED ACCOUNTABILITY. REMINDS HER OF MOTHER——"OH, YOU BELIEVED ME? I'M SORRY"; I'M JUST NOT GOING TO BE HERE. NOT INFUSED WITH ANGER, JUST SWEET REST.

———————

HAD A BREAKDOWN, LOSING IT IN THE WAITING ROOM ABOUT THE POSSIBILITY OF BECOMING PHOBIC ABOUT IVs (WHICH WOULD MAKE HER LIFE HELL GIVEN ALL THE IVs SHE IS BOUND TO GET). FEAR OF FEAR OF PAIN: IVs A FOCAL POINT FOR UNEXPRESSED FEELINGS ABOUT THE WHOLE EXPERIENCE. BUT SOME IT IS THE PUNCTURING OF ONE BODY LAYER AND THEN ANOTHER LAYER OF PAIN IN-SIDE, VEINS ROLLING AROUND RUBBERY AND BRITTLE FROM CHEMO, INESCAP-ABLE, BEING UNABLE TO JUST BE PASSIVE, LET IT WASH OVER HER (HER USUAL RESOURCE FOR DEALING WITH PAIN).

Meanwhile the question of wanting things—being able to want and inhabit the life, the time and loves I have—focuses acutely, and I'm not suprised that the organ where it seems to have taken up dwelling, at this moment, is the fingers. Not that I think of arresting the thread of life as it draws through them, but there's this hunger, which feels like a skin hunger, to handle every rough or silky twist of its passing. I understand it as

> enjoining care to
> the material senses,
> and to making stuff.

TOLD HER ABOUT MY TREADMILL TEST ON FRIDAY ENDING IN THE RECOMMEN-
DATION FOR A CARDIAC CATHETERIZATION.

Yes, I've always been paralyzingly frightened of losing people I love.

At first, when I'd mention such terrors to Shannon I always used to add, "Mustn't that mean I'm teeming with hostile wishes?"

But these were some of the places where "Not necessarily" would be his calming answer. Places where it opened the most possibility: not always to be suspicious of my love and protectiveness for others. The prospect left me gaping. Until gradually I learned to live with it.

But that didn't make me less frightened of losing them. And now the people with whom my empathy's root-deep—Hal, overwhelmingly, but also Michael, my mommy and daddy, David, Stephen, Mary, Mary, Andy, Joe, Meliss, Mandy, José, Jon, Jon, Barbara, Tyler, Lib, Janet, Nina, Nina, Ken, Songmin, Simon, Judy, Maude, Rafael, Renu, Noam, Rosemary, Cynthia, Nahum, Jim, Taddy, Sasha, Cindy, Cathy,

Denise, Josh, Marsha, Mark, Neil, Adam, Jenn, Tim, Laverne, Robert, Daniel, Dan, Katie—I want to say Brian—and, and, and, the big, spreading field of intimacy where love just grows wild—

> it's I threatening
> them now with this crushing freight—
> dread and gravity—

Shannon, threatening me now.

———

WHAT NOW? MY ILLNESS, SUDDEN HOSPITALIZATION, DISRUPT E'S POSITION OF BEING ON ONLY ONE SIDE OF SICK/WELL DIVISION; THROWS HER INTO THE SIDE OF ALSO BEING SOMEONE WHO HAS SOMEONE THEY CARE ABOUT GRAVELY ILL. THIS DISTURBS HER DEVELOPING ACCOMMODATION TO HER OWN ILLNESS. ' SHE HAS ALWAYS FELT IT IS SURVIVORS WHO ARE TO BE PITIED AND THIS BE-COMES ONLY CLEARER AND CLEARER TO HER——EXTREMELY PAINFUL TO THINK ABOUT, BUT IMPORTANT TO.———

———

"I'm loving how pedagogy—the psychology of it—turns up at the center of everything in Tibetan Buddhism. It feels so haimish. Where the difficult part isn't what you need to know, but how to go about really knowing it." Acknowledging the reality, my brother would say. Realizing. Being the slow learner.

It's at Shannon's home I say this—the first time I've been there. I've brought a lunch for us, a heart-healthy one, and he narrates his hospital adventures. He's pale, slow, very shaken, and wearing shorts. Me in that outsize neck brace. One of those melting, autumnal days in the South.

"I'm getting calmed," I tell him, "a bit reassured all around, by how many stories Sogyal Rinpoche tells about gurus dying (calmly or gaily)—their students and intimates sad but, at the same time, very well equipped with a certain soul-seed of that person inside of them." Something they've learned, over a long apprenticeship, to hold as their sense of themselves.

MEANWHILE——*THE TIBETAN BOOK OF THE DEAD.* THE MODEL OF A TRUE AND REVELATORY RELATIONSHIP IS THE GRATITUDE AND TENDERNESS BETWEEN MOTHER AND CHILD / TEACHER AND STUDENT——THE UNIQUE IDEA THAT YOU CAN TELL IF IT'S TRUE BY THE FEELINGS OF TENDERNESS AND GRATITUDE (NOT OEDIPAL-STYLE ENVY, LACK, VIOLENCE)——THAT THIS IS ALSO THE RELATIONSHIP BETWEEN YOU AND THE UNIVERSAL LUMINOSITY WHICH IS (ALSO) YOU. SOME TENSION AS THE MODELS USED ARE INTERSUBJECTIVE (E.G., TEACHER/STUDENT) BUT NONDUAL. BUT E: "NONDUALISM IS MOTHER'S MILK TO ME." THE POSSIBIL- ITY THAT SOME PASSAGE OF DISCONTINUITY LIKE DEATH CAN BE THE OCCASION OF ENLIGHTENMENT, IF YOU DO IT RIGHT, I.E., IF YOU CAN BE IN A PLACE TO RECOGNIZE A LOVE THAT IS YOU AND IS ALSO TOWARD YOU.——THOUGHT OF THE PANDA AS EMBLEMATIC OR SOMEHOW SYMBOLIC OF BUDDHA FOR E——A STYL- IZED FIGURE, NOT INDIVIDUALIZED, SOMETHING THAT ENABLES THE RECOGNI- TION OF PERSONALLY SPECIFIC THINGS IN E.G. HAL AND ME THAT ARE LOVABLE, BUT IT ALSO DEINDIVIDUATES US , MOTHER AND/OR CHILD——SUBJECT AND/OR OBJECT . . .

With my puritanical modernist aesthetic I used to think it was em- barrassing, in a religion like Buddhism, to have images of divinity scattered all over the landscape. It had that whiff of idolatry.

"But I was reading this book, and I happened to look around my liv- ing room, and what was there? Like, twelve or fifteen stuffed pandas and pictures of pandas."

Not because I view them as gods! Not because I believe, even, in God—like my belief mattered.

But because to see them makes me happy. Seeing self and others transmogrified through them—the presence, gravity, and clumsy comedy of these big, inefficient, contented, very endangered bodies. With all their sexual incompetence and soot-black, cookie-cutter ears. It seems so obvious that the more such images there are, the happier.

And it means a lot, to be happy.

It may even mean: to be good. Ungreedy, unattached, unrageful, unignorant. Far different from the pharisaism that says, "I am lucky and happy because I am good," a modest occasional knowledge: I'm good, if I am, because I'm lucky enough to be happy (if I am).

It never seems sensible to pass along moral injunctions. I sometimes think that beyond the Golden Rule,

> the only one that
> matters is this: If you can
> be happy, you should.

———

WONDERS IF SHE IS SHUTTING DOWN SOME AFFECTS, BUT FEELS MORE THAT SHE IS FEELING GOOD, NOT ANXIOUS, READY FOR THESE NEW PROJECTS, TRYING TO HONESTLY RELATE TO THE FUTURE OF HER DEATH. HAD A VERY SOFT, GOOD-FEELING DREAM——THE GROWING WEB OF CONSCIOUSNESS AROUND THE LIMBS, BRANCHES, LEAVES OF TREES ON THE FIRST FEW PAGES OF NEWEST BOOK.

———

TESTS SHOW NO NEW CANCER; TESTS SHOW SAME OLD CANCER. SPINAL PAIN REMAINS BUT SOME LESS. E WORKING ON HOW TO LIVE IN RELATION TO AN INCURABLE, NOT PRESENTLY DEBILITATING ILLNESS. TALKING ABOUT THE NUM- BER OF PEOPLE WHO ASK IF HER NEWS IS GOOD OR BAD——THAT IS NOT A FLEXIBLE OR PRODUCTIVE WAY OF THINKING ABOUT THIS. AN AIM NOT TO HOPE OR FEAR A LOT, NOT LEAD OTHERS TO.

———

Here's a Buddhist meditation I've read about. I can even do it.

It happens in a public place; the substance of it is to recognize that every other person there, one by one, male and female and young and old, has been, in some earlier life, your mother.

Or more likely, in many lives.

And regarding the people one by one, you learn to understand how this could have been so. One by one as you gaze, you can see what kind of mother they were to you; you can see as well, slowly, what kind of a child you were to them.

Over and over and over

you're like Aeneas
encountering a stranger,
Venus, and guessing,

just from the rosy
glow of their neck and their feet,
and their stately step,

though too late, "Surely,
stranger, you are a goddess.
Surely, my mother."

Shy as I am, I'm pretty good at this meditation.

In almost every face I can find the curve of a tenderness, however hidden. The place of a smile or an intelligence—a shared one.

Aeneas: "Why am I never allowed to take your hand in mine, to hear your true voice and speak to you as you really are?"

Even in a skinhead without any lips to speak of; or in a girl who's anxious, anorexic, half crazed with all her narcissistic burden—even from her I can elicit and nurture it, the sense of her possible, beautiful care of me. Indeed, of a compassion; of her imagination, or his.

Of course, with babies it's easy.

In a roomful of my students—I can find it.

———

(No, what makes a wrench
is encountering this part:
I've been their mother,

too! And yet I can't
remember a single thing
about it. It's just

like the frightening
dreams where I know, of course I
do have children, but

have no provision
for them.
        Can't even, if I'm
truthful, remember

where I have left them—
also they all look the same.
Unlike my mothers.)

It's a therapy day and I've driven up to the gray building early for our hour. Early enough to clamber across the parking lot, across the parking lot of the bank next door, across Ninth Street, to ask someone at the BP station on the corner a question about my car.

But the shrubby border between the two parking lots is unexpectedly steep, mulched with its slippery pine needles. Typically clumsy, I tumble, almost fall. Then collecting myself, move on

through the bank's parking
lot with all a fat woman's
disavowing haste.

After my errand, I'm walking back from the gas station when I notice Shannon rounding the corner toward the gray building. He's crossing the bank parking lot ahead of me and doesn't see me.

When Nina and I were in the same high school, she bitterly accused me of embarrassing her by walking around alone looking as if
I was *thinking*. I don't know if that's how Shannon looks; I notice more
the calm buoyancy with which he is able to steer his round, large, light
body, like a float in a Macy's Thanksgiving Day parade.

Even if he is thinking, he's alert to his surroundings. When he
gets near the bottom of the shrubby border, suddenly the balloon
makes a graceful, low dip: I see him gather up from the pavement the
clumps of pine mulch I kicked down as I was teetering on the brink.
Then bobbing up gently, he pats it back into place, his hands briefly
smoothing it in with the other mulch.

Me hanging back, wanting not to be seen.

This little, spied-on
scene: how does it endow me
with hidden treasure?

Why do I feel afterward as if, whatever my frustration or fear, I'm
carrying with me an object of reflection: if I turn inward toward it, it
will make me smile?

I'm wary of such sudden condensations of sweetness, the kind
that, in the past, have made me fall in love.

But I don't resist, either, secretly fingering this enigmatic pebble.
I can't quite figure out what makes its meaning for me.

Diffident, I write to Tim that there may be something inex-
haustibly pleasing in the tight, light knot of space, time, and seeing.
How the small extent of Ninth Street, our wide-skied, midwestern-
feeling little college town, turns into a time-lapse graphic that lets
Shannon occupy the place where I was, encountering my ghost without recognition, unmaking my mistake—me, turning back, seeing it.
And I love that his care for me was not care for *me*.

Tim writes back, "Far from tedious I find the image of Shannon bending over to pick up mulch—the same that you had dislodged, in falling, if I understood you—not knowing it was you who had dislodged it, to have the power of something in De Quincey—or perhaps the film noir version of De Quincey, that I carry around in my head.

"An immediate, involuntary substitution: anonymous shrinks, doing reparative work—in their spare time."

———————

OVER WEEKEND, E GOT A CALL FROM WOMAN SHE HAS KNOWN HERE WHO JUST FOUND OUT SHE TOO HAS BREAST CANCER. E DESCRIBES THIS WOMAN AS AL-READY HAVING A SIGNIFICANT DEPRESSION. SHE DESCRIBES SOMEONE DRIVEN TO KEEP WORKING EVEN IF SHE HAS NO ENJOYMENT IN THE LABOR. TO ME THIS HAS SOMETHING OF THE SOUND OF HOW E USED TO BE IN HER NOT "BEING ABLE TO STOP." SHE REMEMBERS TELLING ME HOW SHE WAITS FOR SOMEONE TO TELL HER SHE CAN "STOP NOW"——E.G., DIE. SHE IMAGINES ME DOING THIS SOMETIME IN THE FUTURE. SHE ALSO TALKS ABOUT HAVING COME TO BE ABLE TO HEAR A VOICE LIKE MY VOICE INSIDE HERSELF WHEN IT IS QUIET THAT SHE CAN TRUST AND HAVE CONFIDENCE IN. I CAN IMAGINE THE VOICE TELLING HER SHE CAN STOP.

Library of Congress Cataloging-in-Publication Data

Sedgwick, Eve Kosofsky.

A dialogue on love / Eve Kosofsky Sedgwick.

p. cm.

ISBN 0-8070-2922-x (cloth)

ISBN 0-8070-2923-8 (pbk.)

1. Sedgwick, Eve Kosofsky. 2. Psychotherapy patients—United
States—Biography. 3. Psychotherapy—Case studies. I. Title.

RC464.S43 1999

616.89'14'092—dc21

[B]   98-53908